MW01125010

NUTRITION and CANCER

Foods, Supplements, and Diet Strategies

This book has been translated into English from the original French version.

DISCLAIMER

The author made every effort to ensure the accuracy and reliability of the information provided in this book, but it is ultimately the responsibility of the reader to exercise discretion and judgment when applying the contents herein. It is highly recommended that readers seek guidance from qualified professionals, including healthcare practitioners or relevant specialists.

Furthermore, the author hereby absolves themselves of any liability for the outcomes that may stem from the use, application, or reliance upon the information provided within this book. This disclaimer encompasses, but is not limited to, any potential loss, injury, or damage – whether direct, indirect, incidental, consequential, or punitive – resulting from actions taken based on the information herein.

By accessing and utilizing the contents of this book, readers acknowledge and agree to indemnify and hold harmless the author from any and all claims, demands, or liabilities that may arise.

NUTRITION and CANCER

Foods, Supplements, and Diet Strategies

SOPHIE DOMINGUES-MONTANARI, PhD

Table of Contents

Prologue to Anti-Cancer Nutrition

Cancer is a reality that affects millions of lives around the world, and its ramifications extend far beyond the disease itself. Understanding the underlying mechanisms of cancer, its risk factors, signs and symptoms to watch for, as well as available treatments, is therefore essential. However, one of the most powerful weapons at our disposal is often overlooked: our diet.

This guide aims to demystify the complex link between nutrition and cancer. We will explore foods that have been identified as warriors against cancer, dietary supplements that can support our health, as well as practical nutritional strategies to integrate these elements into our daily lives. Additionally, we will discuss specific diets that have been studied for their ability to aid in the fight against cancer. We will also discover the importance of the microbiome, this invisible ally residing within us, and how wise dietary choices can strengthen our health from within. Furthermore, we will examine how nutrition can support those facing a cancer diagnosis by helping to alleviate treatment side effects and promoting a better quality of life.

This book not only provides information but also offers practical advice, action plans, recipes, and resources. It is aimed at anyone seeking a better understanding of how their diet can play an essential role in their health.

The Cancer Challenge

Introduction

In recent decades, the prevalence of cancer has significantly increased, affecting millions of lives worldwide. While medical research has progressed, paving the way for new approaches to prevention and treatment, the battle against cancer is far from won. Unfortunately, many individuals continue to face this formidable disease, and the burden of cancer on society remains high.

Before delving into the details of foods, supplements, and nutritional strategies that can help prevent or combat cancer, it is essential to understand the nature of the adversary we are fighting. Cancer is a complex and heterogeneous disease, encompassing a multitude of variants, each with its own characteristics, risk factors, and genetic susceptibilities.

We will therefore address the most common types, such as breast cancer, lung cancer, colon cancer, prostate cancer, as well as other prevalent forms. We will also examine the risk factors, whether genetic, environmental, or lifestyle-related, that can contribute to the development of this disease. Cancer symptoms and diagnostic methods, from mammography to biopsies, will also be explored to aid in early detection, a crucial element for a favorable prognosis.

Regarding treatment, we will discuss various modalities, from surgery to chemotherapy, radiotherapy, immunotherapy, and targeted therapy. Advances in cancer research continue to occur, paving the way for more effective treatments and better survival prospects.

This section will serve as a solid foundation for the rest of our journey through anti-cancer nutrition because by better understanding this disease in all its facets, we can arm ourselves with knowledge to make informed decisions about our health and well-being.

Understanding Cancer

Cancer is a condition that often evokes serious concerns. But what exactly is cancer? Why is this disease so feared? To better understand this, we will explore the underlying aspects and explain what happens in our bodies when cancer develops.

The World of Cells

Let's start by taking a close look at our cells, the fundamental units of our organism. They are so small that they can only be seen under a microscope, but they are incredibly numerous: our organs and tissues are made up of billions of cells.

Each cell has a specific role to play. Imagine your body as a large metropolis, where cells are inhabitants working for the proper functioning of the city. For example, skin cells protect our body against external aggressions or infections, liver cells help us digest food, while brain cells allow us to think and make decisions.

For our body to function properly, our cells must divide regularly. This means they reproduce to replace old or damaged cells. This process of cell division is strictly regulated.

However, an error can occur during cell division, and a cell may undergo mutations, meaning changes in its DNA (the genetic information that controls its function). This can be caused by external factors such as smoking or exposure to ultraviolet rays from the sun, or by internal factors such as random errors or cell aging.

The Emergence of Cancer

When a cell undergoes mutations that affect its DNA, it can begin to behave abnormally. Thus, instead of dividing in a regular and controlled manner, it may start to divide uncontrollably and form a mass of abnormal cells called a tumor.

It is important to note that not all tumors are cancerous. Therefore, tumors can be classified into two main categories based on their behavior: benign tumors, which are usually not dangerous, and malignant tumors, or cancerous ones.

Several factors influence this distinction:

- **Cellular differentiation:** Cells forming a benign tumor are usually well-differentiated, meaning they resemble their original cells and function similarly. In contrast, malignant tumors are often less differentiated and exhibit abnormal cellular characteristics.

- **Uncontrolled cell growth:** Benign tumors tend to have slower cell growth and are typically surrounded by a fibrous capsule that confines them. Malignant tumors are characterized by rapid cell growth and can invade surrounding tissues.

- **Metastasis:** The primary distinction between benign and malignant tumors lies in their ability to metastasize. Indeed, malignant tumors have the ability to leave the original tumor, circulate through the blood or lymph, and settle in other organs or tissues, where they form new tumors. Metastases are thus like "colonies" of cancer cells in other parts of our body. They disrupt the normal functioning of these organs and can cause serious health problems. Benign tumors, on the other hand, generally do not spread.

So why do some tumors remain benign while others become malignant? Many factors play a role, including:

- **Genetic factors:** Genetic alterations and mutations can contribute to the development of malignant tumors. Some malignant tumors are associated with specific mutations that promote their invasive behavior.

- **Tumor microenvironment:** The microenvironment surrounding the tumor, including the immune system and growth factors, can influence its behavior. A microenvironment conducive to tumor growth can promote malignancy.

- **Location:** The location of the tumor can also play a role. Some regions of the body tolerate tumors better, while others may lead to serious complications even with benign tumors.

- **Exposure to risk factors:** Exposure to risk factors such as smoking, radiation exposure, an unbalanced diet, and other environmental influences can increase the risk of developing malignant tumors.

The Different Types of Cancer

It's important to understand that cancer can arise in various parts of our bodies, giving rise to many distinct cancers. Each of them is characterized by the type of cell from which it develops. For example, breast cancer originates in breast cells, lung cancer in lung cells, and so on. The prognosis depends on many factors, including the stage at the time of diagnosis, the aggressiveness of the disease, and the response to treatment.

Breast Cancer

Breast cancer is the most commonly diagnosed cancer among women. Although the mortality rate has been declining since the 1990s, the incidence of this cancer continues to rise.

This type of cancer develops in breast cells and can manifest as nodules or tumors in the breast. Although the disease can be asymptomatic in its early stages, there are several symptoms that may alert women and require medical consultation:

- Palpable mass or lump in the breast or armpit.

- Changes in the size, shape, or appearance of the breast, including swelling, thinning, or distortion.

- Persistent pain in the breast or armpit.

- Abnormal nipple discharge outside of pregnancy or breastfeeding.

- Abnormally wrinkled, red, or inflamed breast skin.

Risk factors for breast cancer include age (increased risk after 50 years), family and personal history of breast cancer, genetic mutations (such as BRCA1 and BRCA2 genes), prolonged exposure to estrogen (e.g., early menarche, late menopause), lifestyle (overweight after menopause, alcohol consumption, lack of physical activity), and factors like previous radiotherapy. High breast density can also increase the risk.

Mammography remains one of the most effective methods for detecting breast cancer at an early stage, long before the onset of obvious symptoms, when the tumor is still small and localized. Screening guidelines may vary from country to country, but generally, women are encouraged to undergo regular mammograms from the age of 50, depending on their individual risk factors and local medical guidelines.

The importance of regular breast cancer screening cannot be overstated. It allows doctors to promptly initiate appropriate treatment, often with less invasive techniques, resulting in much better prospects for recovery.

Lung Cancer

Lung cancer is one of the most common and serious forms of cancer in both men and women. Although progress has been made in treatment and early detection, lung cancer remains one of the deadliest cancers.

This type of cancer primarily develops in the cells of the bronchi but can also affect other areas of the lungs. Symptoms are often not evident in the early stages of the disease, making early diagnosis difficult. However, some signs should raise concern:

- Persistent or worsening cough.
- Chest pain that does not go away and may be worsened by deep breathing, coughing, or laughing.

- Shortness of breath or difficulty breathing.

- Hoarseness or changes in voice.

- Blood in the sputum.

The main culprit of lung cancer is smoking, but other risk factors may include exposure to certain toxic substances such as asbestos, radiation, air pollution, and certain viruses.

Due to the often asymptomatic nature of lung cancer in its early stages, screening is crucial for detection at an earlier and more treatable stage, especially for individuals at high risk. It may involve X-rays and low-dose CT scans.

Colorectal Cancer

Colorectal cancer is one of the most common types of cancer, affecting thousands of people each year. This disease particularly affects the mucous membrane of the colon or rectum.

Symptoms can vary and are not always obvious in the early stages. However, some signs should be monitored:

- Changes in bowel habits, such as persistent diarrhea or constipation.

- Presence of blood in the stool or black stools.

- Persistent abdominal pain or cramps.

- Feeling of incomplete bowel emptying.

- Unexplained weight loss.

Early screening for colorectal cancer is crucial as it allows the disease to be detected at a stage where it is more easily treatable. The most common screening test is colonoscopy, which allows examination of the inside of the colon and detection of polyps or other abnormalities that could be cancerous.

Risk factors for colorectal cancer include age (risk increases after 50 years), family history of colorectal cancer, certain inflammatory bowel conditions, a diet low in fiber and high in fats, as well as smoking and excessive alcohol consumption.

Prostate Cancer

Prostate cancer is one of the most common cancers in older men, especially after the age of 50. This type of cancer develops in the prostate, a small gland located in the male pelvis, which plays a key role in the male reproductive system.

Symptoms of prostate cancer can be nonspecific and often do not manifest in the early stages. However, some signs should be noted:

- Difficulty urinating, including weak or interrupted urine flow.
- Frequent need to urinate, particularly at night.
- Presence of blood in the urine or semen.
- Pain or discomfort in the pelvic region.
- Pain during ejaculation.

Early detection is crucial for managing prostate cancer. It is typically done through a blood test measuring the level of prostate-specific antigen (PSA), although controversial due to risks of overdiagnosis, or a digital rectal examination.

Risk factors include age, family history, as well as certain environmental factors.

Skin Cancer

Skin cancer is one of the types of cancer that is steadily increasing in many countries.

It mainly presents in two forms:

- **Carcinoma:** It develops from the cells of the epidermis (the superficial skin cells). There are two main types of carcinomas: basal cell carcinoma, which is the most common and develops slowly, and squamous cell carcinoma, which is less common but can be more aggressive. Carcinomas rarely spread to other parts of the body.

- **Melanoma:** It is less common but more dangerous than carcinomas. Melanoma originates in melanocytes, the cells responsible for skin pigmentation. It tends to spread more rapidly to other parts of the body, making it a more formidable skin cancer.

Symptoms vary by type but may include:

- Changes in the appearance of the skin, such as the formation of new spots or changes in existing moles.

- Wounds that do not heal.

- Skin lesions that itch, bleed, or are painful.

- Appearance of bumps or spots that are pink, red, white, blue, or black on the skin.

- Moles that change in size, shape, color, or texture.

Early detection is essential. It is recommended to regularly examine your skin for any changes and to consult a dermatologist if in doubt. Photos can be taken to track the evolution of moles or other skin lesions.

More than 85% of these cases are attributable to exposure to ultraviolet (UV) radiation. Thus, preventing skin cancer is possible by adopting sun protection measures, such as using broad-spectrum sunscreen, wearing protective clothing, and limiting sun exposure, especially during the hottest hours. It is also advisable to avoid the use of tanning beds.

It is important to note that the types of cancer presented here are among the most commonly diagnosed, but there are many others. Each type of cancer has its own risk factors, screening methods, and specific prevention strategies. Understanding these differences is essential for better combating this complex and varied disease.

Worldwide Cancer Incidence

The statistics regarding cancer are alarming, highlighting the magnitude of this public health challenge on a global scale, with notable variations between regions and disparities in terms of prevalence and mortality.

Global Statistics

In 2020, according to data from the World Health Organization, nearly 18.1 million new cases of cancer were diagnosed worldwide, resulting in 9.9 million deaths.

It is estimated that in 2023, the most common type of cancer globally was breast cancer, accounting for 12.5% of new cases, making it the most diagnosed cancer in women. Lung cancer came in second, comprising 12.2% of new cases, highlighting the continued impact of smoking and exposure to air pollution. In third place, colorectal cancer was responsible for 10.7% of new diagnoses, emphasizing the importance of prevention and early detection.

The data also reveal a troubling trend of increasing incidence and mortality related to cancer. This increase can be attributed to various factors, including population growth, aging populations, unhealthy lifestyles, exposure to harmful environmental factors, and lack of access to quality healthcare in some regions of the world.

Regional Disparities

Cancer is a widespread disease worldwide. However, here are some regions and countries that are particularly affected:

- **Industrialized Western regions:** Countries in Western Europe, North America (United States and Canada), and Oceania (Australia and New Zealand) have relatively high cancer rates due to factors such as smoking, alcohol consumption, a diet rich in fats and processed meats, as well as other risk factors associated with modern lifestyles.

- **East Asia:** Some countries in East Asia, such as Japan, South Korea, and China, have experienced a significant increase in cancer incidence, partly due to changes in dietary and lifestyle habits, rapid urbanization, and exposure to environmental factors.

- **South Asia:** India and some other countries in South Asia are experiencing an increasing prevalence of cancer due to the large population and challenges related to access to healthcare, awareness, and prevention.

- **Sub-Saharan Africa:** This region of the world has lower cancer rates than some industrialized regions, but faces challenges in early diagnosis, treatment, and access to healthcare, which can contribute to higher cancer mortality.

- **Latin America:** Some countries in Latin America have high cancer rates, especially concerning tobacco and alcohol-related cancers. Cervical cancer is also a concern in certain regions of Latin America.

It is important to note that cancer rates can vary significantly within a country or region depending on various socio-economic and geographical factors.

Factors of Disparity

Health inequalities, including those related to cancer, are a complex and multidimensional issue. These inequalities can stem from various factors, including gender, ethnic origin, and socioeconomic conditions. Let's explore how these factors can influence cancer incidence, diagnosis, treatment, and prognosis.

- **Gender-related inequalities:** Men and women may be affected by different types of cancer disproportionately. For example, breast cancer is primarily associated with women, while prostate cancer is common among men. Gender inequalities can also play a role in access to healthcare. Sometimes, women face social, economic, or cultural barriers that limit their access to screenings and treatments.

- **Ethnicity-related inequalities:** Different ethnic communities may have varying rates of cancer due to various factors, including genetic differences, lifestyle habits, and access to healthcare. Ethnic disparities can also influence how patients are diagnosed and treated. It is essential to consider these differences to provide quality and equitable care.

- **Socioeconomic-related inequalities:** Socioeconomic conditions, such as income, education, and access to resources, play a significant role in cancer inequalities. Individuals from disadvantaged socioeconomic backgrounds often have an increased risk of developing certain types of cancer. Financial barriers, lack of health insurance, and economic instability can lead to limited access to healthcare, screening, and quality treatment.

It is imperative to recognize these inequalities and take steps to reduce them. This includes developing public health policies aimed at promoting equal access to healthcare, raising further awareness about cancer prevention in vulnerable communities, and conducting research to better understand the underlying factors contributing to these inequalities.

Survival Rates

Survival rates play a crucial role in understanding the severity of a disease like cancer. They are influenced by a multitude of factors, including social and economic inequalities, as well as the type and stage of cancer at the time of diagnosis.

The significant variations noted in survival rates underscore the importance of early detection and the fight against health disparities. Thus, it can be observed that some cancers have more favorable prognoses than others. For example, melanoma and prostate cancer have relatively high 5-year survival rates in France, averaging around 90-95%. These encouraging results are often attributed to several factors, such as advances in early detection, effective treatments, and increased awareness of these diseases.

However, other types of cancer present much lower survival rates. For instance, pancreatic cancer, lung cancer, and glioblastoma, an aggressive form of brain cancer, have much darker 5-year survival rates. These cancers are often diagnosed at an advanced stage, significantly reducing the chances of cure.

Health inequalities also play a crucial role in the disparity of survival rates. Individuals from disadvantaged socioeconomic groups often have limited access to healthcare, which can delay diagnosis and treatment, thus worsening already unfavorable prognoses.

To combat these inequalities and improve survival rates for all cancer patients, it is necessary to promote awareness, early screening, equitable access to healthcare, and continuous research into new treatments.

Rising Trends

The rising trends in cancer are a concerning issue, closely linked to several significant factors shaping our modern society.

One of these trends is related to the aging population. With improvements in healthcare and living conditions, life expectancy is increasing, which is excellent news in itself. However, this natural increase in longevity is accompanied by a rise in the number of cancer cases. Indeed, the risk of developing cancer significantly increases with age, so the more elderly people there are in the population, the more cancer cases there will be.

Rapid urbanization is another major factor contributing to this upward trend. Changes in our lifestyles, especially in urban areas, have a significant impact. Modern lifestyles are often characterized by unhealthy eating habits, rich in processed foods, reduced physical activity due to sedentary lifestyles associated with office jobs and motorized transportation, and high stress levels. All these factors are associated with an increased risk of developing cancer. Therefore, promoting healthy lifestyles in urban environments is crucial to reversing this trend.

Regarding exposure to carcinogens, many environmental factors contribute to the increase in cancer cases. Air, water, and soil pollution, as well as exposure to toxic chemicals in our food and consumer products, play a crucial role. Additionally, smoking remains one of the leading causes of cancer worldwide. Awareness campaigns and efforts to reduce tobacco consumption are essential to counteracting this upward trend.

In conclusion, the fight against cancer requires international cooperation, ongoing commitment, and sustained attention to all aspects of prevention, screening, treatment, and patient support. Only by combining these efforts can we hope to reduce the devastating impact of cancer worldwide.

Risk Factors

Behavioral Factors

Understanding how our daily behaviors can influence our risk of cancer is essential for making informed health decisions. Smoking, alcohol consumption, and sedentary lifestyle are among the most studied behaviors in relation to cancer, and they play a major role in our overall health.

Smoking

Smoking has long been identified as one of the most significant risk factors associated with many types of cancer, including lung, mouth, throat, and bladder cancer. This close relationship between tobacco and cancer is supported by decades of scientific research.

Tobacco smoke is a complex concoction of thousands of chemicals, including many notorious carcinogenic substances such as tar, benzene, formaldehyde, and nickel, to name a few. When smokers inhale these toxic compounds, they penetrate deep into the respiratory tract, reaching the lungs and the oral mucosa. There, carcinogenic substances damage the DNA of cells, causing mutations that can trigger faulty cellular mechanisms, thus promoting the anarchic growth of cancer cells. This is how smoking becomes the starting point for many forms of cancer.

Lung cancer, an aggressive and often deadly disease, is the most notorious example of the devastating impact of smoking. Tobacco smoke alters lung cells, transforming them into malignant tumors that are difficult to treat.

In addition to lung cancer, smoking is also closely linked to other forms of cancer. For example, mouth and throat cancers are often observed in smokers because tobacco smoke can cause precancerous lesions in these regions, which then evolve into malignant tumors. Furthermore, inhaled smoke passes through the lungs and comes into contact with the throat mucosa, thus exposing these tissues to carcinogenic agents.

Bladder cancer is another cancer strongly influenced by smoking. Toxic chemicals present in tobacco smoke are filtered by the kidneys and excreted in urine. As a result, the bladder is repeatedly exposed to these harmful substances, significantly increasing the risk of developing bladder cancer.

Quitting smoking can significantly reduce the risk of smoking-related cancer. Damaged cells have the ability to gradually repair themselves when exposure to tobacco smoke ceases. The earlier a person quits smoking, the greater the chances of reducing their risk of developing cancer. This underscores the crucial importance of smoking cessation as a cancer prevention measure.

Alcohol Consumption

Alcohol consumption is an aspect of our social and cultural lives that can sometimes be underestimated in terms of its impact on health, especially regarding the risk of cancer. However, it is essential to understand that alcohol is a well-established risk factor for several types of cancer, and its role in the development of the disease should not be ignored.

Alcohol contains ethanol, a chemical substance that can damage cells and tissues in the body. When we consume alcohol, ethanol is metabolized by our liver into acetaldehyde, a highly toxic and carcinogenic substance. Acetaldehyde can cause DNA mutations and cellular damage, thereby creating an environment conducive to the formation of cancer cells.

Among the types of cancer most closely linked to alcohol consumption are mouth, throat, esophagus, liver, colon, and breast cancer. The risk of cancer increases in a dose-dependent manner, meaning that the more alcohol a person consumes, the higher their risk of developing cancer. Even light to moderate alcohol consumption can significantly increase the risk of cancer.

It is important to note that the type of alcohol consumed does not have significant relevance in terms of cancer risk. Whether one drinks beer, wine, or spirits, they all contain ethanol, and it is this substance that is responsible for cellular damage.

Preventing alcohol-related cancer primarily involves reducing the amount of alcohol consumed. While total abstinence is the best option in terms of prevention, it is understandable that this may be difficult for some. In this case, it is essential to limit alcohol consumption to safe levels. Health guidelines typically recommend not exceeding one alcoholic drink per day for women and two for men.

Sedentary Lifestyle

Another major risk factor often underestimated in cancer development is sedentary behavior, which refers to a lack of physical activity. Our modern lifestyles, characterized by long hours spent sitting in front of computer or television screens, driving instead of walking or cycling, and a lack of regular exercise, have contributed to an alarming increase in sedentary behavior worldwide. However, this inactivity can have serious health consequences, including an increased risk of cancer.

One of the mechanisms by which sedentary behavior can promote cancer is its close relationship with obesity. Sedentary individuals tend to burn fewer calories than those leading an active lifestyle, which can lead to excessive weight gain. Obesity, in turn, is a major risk factor for many types of cancer, including breast, uterine, colon, kidney, and liver cancer. Fat cells produce hormones and inflammatory cytokines that can create a pro-inflammatory environment in the body, promoting the growth of cancer cells.

Furthermore, sedentary behavior can also lead to detrimental metabolic changes. Inactive individuals are more likely to develop insulin resistance, a metabolic disorder that can lead to increased insulin levels in the blood. Insulin is a hormone that promotes cell growth, and high levels of insulin can create an environment conducive to the proliferation of cancer cells.

Fortunately, there is a simple and effective solution to reduce the risk of cancer associated with sedentary behavior: regular exercise. Even moderate physical activity, such as swimming, cycling, or gardening, can have a positive impact on health. This can also include regular walks, taking the stairs instead of the elevator, or engaging in active leisure activities such as dancing or yoga. Exercise helps maintain a healthy body weight, strengthens the immune system, and reduces inflammation. Additionally, it can help regulate insulin levels, reducing the risk of tumor development.

Complex Interactions

When examining cancer risk factors such as smoking, sedentary behavior, and alcohol consumption, it becomes evident that these behaviors are not isolated from each other. On the contrary, they often interact in complex ways, creating a cumulative impact on the risk of developing the disease.

Take smoking, for example. Smoking is associated with an increased risk of lung, mouth, throat, and bladder cancer, among others. However, smoking is not limited to the act of smoking a cigarette. It is often accompanied by other harmful habits, such as alcohol consumption and an unhealthy diet. Smokers sometimes tend to neglect their diet, opting for foods high in saturated fats, sugar, and salt. This unbalanced diet can contribute to obesity, chronic inflammation, and other cancer risk factors.

On the other hand, sedentary behavior can also be linked to smoking. People who smoke sometimes tend to be less physically active, which can exacerbate the harmful effects of tobacco on their health. Lack of exercise can contribute to weight gain, poor cardiovascular health, and a reduced ability of the body to defend against cancer cells. Thus, the combination of sedentary behavior and smoking can create an environment particularly conducive to cancer development.

Alcohol consumption also comes into play in this complex equation. Alcohol can be a common way to socialize, often associated with festive events or social occasions. During these times, it is common to consume high-calorie, high-fat foods to accompany alcohol. Moreover, alcohol can lower inhibitions, sometimes leading to less healthy food choices. Thus, alcohol consumption can reinforce the negative effects of smoking and sedentary behavior on cancer risk.

It becomes evident, then, that these health risk behaviors should not be viewed in isolation but rather as interconnected elements of an overall lifestyle. Adopting a healthy lifestyle overall, which includes quitting smoking, reducing alcohol consumption, maintaining a balanced diet, and increasing physical activity, is essential to significantly reduce the risk of cancer.

In conclusion, our daily behaviors have a significant impact on our cancer risk, and understanding the complex interactions between health risk behaviors is essential to effectively combat cancer. It allows us to make informed decisions about our lifestyle and reduce the risk of developing this devastating disease.

Genetic Factors

Understanding how our family history and genes can influence our risk of cancer is crucial for a personalized approach to prevention. These factors can play a major role in cancer predisposition.

The Role of Genetics

The role of genetics in cancer development is a complex and fascinating issue. Our genetic code, contained within DNA, significantly influences our susceptibility to various types of cancer. However, it is important to note that genetics is just one component of a broader picture that also includes environmental and behavioral factors.

At the core of the relationship between genetics and cancer are genetic mutations. Mutations are alterations in DNA that can occur spontaneously or be inherited. Some genetic mutations significantly increase the risk of cancer. For example, mutations in the BRCA1 and BRCA2 genes are associated with an increased risk of breast and ovarian cancer, while mutations in the TP53 gene are linked to an increased risk of several types of cancer, including breast, brain, and bone cancers.

Family history of cancer can be an important indicator of genetic predisposition to cancer. If close family members have been affected by a certain type of cancer, it may suggest genetic transmission. Individuals with a family history of cancer may be encouraged to undergo genetic testing to identify potential mutations. Early detection of these mutations can allow for appropriate medical management and preventive measures to reduce the risk.

It is essential to understand that genetics does not operate in isolation. Environmental and behavioral factors interact with our genes to influence our risk of cancer. For example, a person with a genetic predisposition to lung cancer may be more vulnerable to the carcinogenic effects of smoking. Similarly, a healthy diet, regular exercise, and other lifestyle choices can modulate the effects of genetics on cancer risk.

Research in cancer genetics is progressing rapidly. Scientists are identifying more and more genes associated with specific types of cancer, leading to a better understanding of underlying mechanisms. This knowledge is valuable for the development of targeted treatments and personalized therapies.

Genetic Counseling

For individuals with a family history of cancer, oncogenetic counseling can be an essential tool for assessing genetic risk, understanding implications, and making informed decisions about cancer prevention and screening.

When consulting a counselor, the first step is to assess your genetic risk. This is done by examining your family history of cancer, particularly the types of cancer that have affected your relatives and the age at which these cancers were diagnosed. The genetic counselor will also gather information about your own medical history and lifestyle.

Based on this assessment, the genetic counselor may recommend appropriate genetic testing. These tests aim to identify specific mutations that may increase your cancer risk. For example, if your family has a history of breast cancer, BRCA gene testing may be recommended. The results of these tests can provide crucial information about your susceptibility to cancer.

Once the results of genetic testing are available, the genetic counselor will explain their implications in detail. If a genetic mutation is detected, you will discuss prevention and screening options.

Genetic counseling also provides essential support. Receiving a diagnosis of a cancer-associated genetic mutation can be a challenging experience. Genetic counselors are trained to help individuals and families cope with this reality, answer their questions, and provide psychological support.

It is important to note that genetic counseling is based on principles of professional ethics and confidentiality. Genetic information is highly confidential, and genetic counselors are required to adhere to the strictest ethical standards to protect the privacy of their patients.

Prevention and Management

When a genetic predisposition to cancer is identified, it becomes imperative to implement personalized prevention measures to reduce the risk of developing the disease. These measures are tailored to each individual based on their family history, identified genetic mutations, and other risk factors. Here's how cancer prevention and risk management can be approached in a personalized manner:

- **Personalized Screening:** One of the pillars of prevention for individuals at genetic risk is personalized screening. This means that individuals may undergo more frequent medical exams and advanced screening to detect any early signs of cancer. For example, a person with genetic mutations associated with breast cancer may benefit from more frequent mammograms and breast MRIs to detect any potential changes.

- **Preventive Surgeries:** In some cases, preventive surgeries may be recommended to significantly reduce the risk of cancer. This may include preventive mastectomy to reduce the risk of breast cancer in high-risk women, or preventive colectomy to reduce the risk of colorectal cancer. These decisions are made in close collaboration with patients and their medical team.

- **Lifestyle Modifications:** Lifestyle modification is also an essential element of cancer prevention. For individuals at genetic risk, it may be particularly important to reduce other cancer risk factors. Healthcare professionals can provide specific advice on how to adopt a healthier lifestyle.

- **Regular Medical Follow-up:** Regular medical follow-up is crucial to ensure that prevention measures are working effectively. Patients should maintain open communication with their medical team, participate in recommended screenings, and report any changes or suspicious symptoms.

In conclusion, family history and genes play a complex role in cancer risk. While these factors may increase vulnerability, they do not necessarily determine destiny. A thorough understanding of these influences can enable proactive and personalized healthcare management, to reduce the risk of cancer and promote long-term well-being.

Environmental Factors

Understanding how exposure to toxic substances and pollution can influence the development of cancer is essential for minimizing risks to our health. Indeed, our environment can play a major role in the occurrence of this disease.

Toxic Substances

The impact of toxic substances on cancer risk is a concerning issue in our modern society. Many dangerous chemicals are present in our environment, and their exposure can have serious consequences for human health. Here's how these toxic substances can increase the risk of cancer:

- **Industrial Chemicals:** Industrial chemicals are ubiquitous in our daily lives, whether in construction materials, cleaning products, plastics, or other manufactured goods. Some of these products contain potentially carcinogenic chemical compounds, such as polycyclic aromatic hydrocarbons (PAHs) and organic solvents. People exposed to these chemicals in the workplace or at home may have an increased risk of cancer, especially if they do not take necessary precautions to minimize their exposure.

- **Pesticides:** Pesticides are used in agriculture to protect crops from pests. However, many pesticides contain potentially carcinogenic substances. Farmers and people living near agricultural areas may be exposed to these chemicals through inhalation, skin contact, or accidental ingestion. Studies have shown links between pesticide exposure and an increased risk of certain types of cancer, including breast, prostate, and brain cancer.

- **Heavy Metals:** Heavy metals such as lead, mercury, cadmium, and arsenic are contaminants present in water, soil, and air. These metals can accumulate in the body over time and cause significant damage. For example, lead is associated with kidney cancer, mercury with lung cancer, and cadmium with prostate cancer. Exposure to these heavy metals can occur through consumption of contaminated water or food, as well as inhalation of toxic dust.

- **Carcinogenic Substances:** In addition to industrial chemicals, pesticides, and heavy metals, there are many other carcinogenic substances present in our daily environment. This includes compounds in tobacco smoke, atmospheric pollutants, chemicals in common consumer products, and even substances in certain processed foods. Chronic exposure to these substances can gradually increase the risk of cancer over time.

To reduce the risk of cancer related to exposure to toxic substances, it is essential to take preventive measures. This may include adopting workplace safety practices for workers exposed to chemicals, reducing the use of toxic household chemicals, and raising awareness about indoor and outdoor air quality.

Air Pollution

Air pollution has become one of the most serious environmental threats of our time, with devastating implications for human health, particularly concerning cancer. This insidious form of pollution, caused by emissions from vehicles, industrial factories, power plants, and other sources, poses a major health risk.

One of the most concerning aspects of air pollution lies in the fine particles and chemical compounds it contains. These tiny particles, invisible to the naked eye, are small enough to be deeply inhaled into the lungs. There, they cause inflammation and severe cellular damage. Some of these particles contain harmful chemical compounds, including carcinogens, which can damage the DNA of lung cells and other tissues.

The link between air pollution and lung cancer is particularly alarming. Lung cancer is one of the deadliest types of cancer worldwide, and chronic exposure to atmospheric pollutants significantly contributes to its increasing incidence. Airborne carcinogens, such as benzene, formaldehyde, and polycyclic aromatic hydrocarbons (PAHs), are released into the atmosphere by vehicle emissions and industrial facilities. When inhaled, these chemicals can damage the DNA of lung cells, causing mutations that promote the growth of cancer cells.

Air pollution is not limited to lung cancer. It is also associated with other forms of cancer, including bladder, breast, prostate, and even brain cancer. Additionally, long-term exposure to air pollution can have systemic effects on health, increasing the risk of cardiovascular diseases, chronic respiratory diseases, and neurological disorders.

To reduce the risk of cancer related to air pollution, preventive measures are essential. This includes promoting cleaner modes of transportation, reducing industrial emissions, adopting cleaner energy production technologies, and strengthening environmental regulations. Individually, people can contribute by limiting their exposure to air pollution by avoiding heavily polluted areas, using indoor air filters, and supporting initiatives aimed at reducing atmospheric pollution.

Water Pollution

The quality of the water we consume is of paramount importance to our health, but unfortunately, many sources of drinking water around the world are contaminated with harmful substances. Exposure to contaminants in drinking water, such as heavy metals, industrial chemicals, and organic pollutants, can have serious consequences for our well-being, including an increased risk of digestive system cancers.

For instance, certain heavy metals like lead, mercury, and cadmium can find their way into drinking water due to human activity, including industrial discharges and the use of lead pipes. These metals are toxic to the human body and can accumulate in bodily tissues. Prolonged exposure to low levels of these metals through drinking water has been associated with an increased risk of cancer, particularly in the digestive system.

Additionally, industrial chemicals such as solvents, volatile organic compounds (VOCs), and pesticides can contaminate drinking water due to accidental spills, leaks, or agricultural practices. Some of these chemicals have been identified as potential carcinogens. For example, exposure to tetrachloroethylene (perchloroethylene), a solvent used in dry cleaning, can increase the risk of esophageal cancer.

Epidemiological studies have established a link between consumption of contaminated water and an increased risk of esophageal, stomach, liver, pancreatic, and colon cancers. Moreover, in regions where drinking water is contaminated with arsenic, a heavy metal naturally present in the soil, there is an increased risk of bladder, skin, and digestive system cancers.

Preventing exposure to contaminated water is essential to reduce the risk of digestive system cancer and other health problems. This may involve implementing stricter regulations on water quality, regular monitoring of drinking water quality, decontaminating water using appropriate technologies, and raising public awareness about the risks associated with contaminated water.

Individually, you can take steps to protect your health by using a home water filtration system to remove potential contaminants, avoiding consumption of water from suspect sources, and supporting water conservation efforts and environmental protection to prevent water pollution at the source.

Work Conditions

The link between work conditions and the risk of cancer is an important concern in occupational health. Some professions expose workers to carcinogenic substances, which can significantly increase their risk of developing cancer. Understanding these risks and implementing appropriate workplace safety regulations is essential to protect workers' health.

Asbestos is one of the most notorious examples of carcinogenic substances in the workplace. Before being banned in many countries, asbestos was widely used in construction and industry for its fireproof and insulating properties. However, inhaling asbestos fibers can cause a variety of cancers, including pleural mesothelioma, a rare but aggressive cancer that develops in the membranes surrounding the lungs.

Workers exposed to asbestos, such as construction workers, plumbers, and electricians, were particularly at risk. Strict asbestos regulations, including its removal and safe containment, were put in place to minimize these occupational risks.

Additionally, many industries, including the chemical industry, the oil and gas industry, and manufacturing, use potentially hazardous chemicals in their production processes. Some of these chemicals are classified as carcinogens and can increase the risk of cancer in exposed workers.

For example, exposure to chemicals such as benzene, formaldehyde, and vinyl chloride may be linked to an increased risk of leukemia, nasopharyngeal cancer, lung cancer, and liver cancer.

To minimize the risks of cancer related to work conditions, preventive measures are essential:

- **Work Safety Regulations:** Governments and regulatory bodies must implement strict regulations to control the use of carcinogenic substances in the workplace. This includes permissible exposure limits, engineering controls to reduce the emission of hazardous substances, and personal protective equipment for workers.

- **Training and Awareness:** Employers should provide adequate training to workers on the health risks associated with their work, as well as on preventive measures and safety protocols to follow.

- **Health Monitoring:** Workers exposed to carcinogenic substances should receive regular health monitoring to detect any early signs of cancer. This may include regular medical examinations, blood tests, and chest X-rays, depending on the nature of the exposure.

Signs and Symptoms

Warning Signs

It is essential to recognize the signs and symptoms of cancer because an early diagnosis can make a huge difference in the chances of successful treatment. Although these symptoms can be caused by other health problems, it is important to take them seriously.

Digestive Symptoms

Digestive symptoms can indicate the presence of a malignant disease in the digestive system. It is important to note that such symptoms are not always synonymous with cancer, but they should nevertheless be taken seriously and evaluated by a healthcare professional. These symptoms may vary depending on the type and location of cancer, but some common signs include:

- **Changes in bowel habits:** Significant changes in the frequency of bowel movements, stool consistency (persistent constipation or diarrhea), or the sensation of incomplete bowel emptying may be a sign of colorectal cancer.

- **Rectal bleeding:** The presence of blood in stools or unexplained rectal bleeding should be carefully evaluated, as it may indicate colorectal or anal cancer.

- **Persistent abdominal pain:** Abdominal pain or cramps that persist for an extended period, without an obvious cause such as common gastrointestinal disorders, may be an indicator of stomach, pancreatic, liver, or intestinal cancer.

- **Unexplained weight loss:** Significant weight loss without changes in dietary habits or physical activity may be a symptom of various types of digestive cancer, including stomach, esophageal, or pancreatic cancer.

- **Bloating and abdominal distension:** Persistent bloating, a feeling of fullness after small amounts of food, or abnormal abdominal distension may indicate stomach or intestinal cancer.

- **Difficulty swallowing:** Dysphagia, or difficulty swallowing, may result from esophageal cancer or other tumors that obstruct the passage of food.

- **Persistent gastroesophageal reflux (GERD):** Frequent and persistent acid reflux may be associated with esophageal cancer, especially if accompanied by chest pain or difficulty swallowing.

- **Jaundice:** Yellowing of the skin and eyes (jaundice) may be a sign of liver, gallbladder, or bile duct cancer.

Anyone experiencing any of these symptoms should consult a doctor for an accurate diagnosis. Early screening for digestive cancer can significantly improve the chances of effective treatment and recovery. Therefore, it is recommended not to ignore these warning signs and to seek appropriate medical evaluation.

Respiratory Symptoms

Respiratory symptoms can indicate the presence of a malignant tumor in the respiratory tract or organs such as the lungs or throat. They vary depending on the type of cancer and its location, but here are some common signs to watch out for:

- **Persistent Cough:** A cough that lasts for more than a few weeks, especially if accompanied by coughing up blood, chest pain, or difficulty breathing, may indicate lung cancer.

- **Shortness of Breath:** If you experience unusual shortness of breath, especially in the absence of exercise or physical exertion, it may be a sign of lung cancer or airway obstruction.

- **Changes in Voice:** Persistent changes in voice, such as hoarseness or a hoarse voice, may be related to throat, vocal cord, or tracheal cancer.

- **Chest Pain:** Persistent chest pain, sometimes associated with coughing or difficulty breathing, may indicate the presence of a lung tumor or other thoracic cancers.

- **Coughing Up Blood:** The presence of blood in sputum, even in small amounts, requires immediate medical evaluation, as it may be a sign of respiratory tract or lung cancer.

- **Frequent Respiratory Infections:** If you frequently suffer from respiratory infections such as pneumonia or bronchitis, it may be related to obstruction caused by a tumor.

- **Swelling of the Neck or Face:** Swelling of the neck or face may result from pressure exerted by a tumor on the upper respiratory tract and should be examined by a doctor.

- **Unexplained Weight Loss:** Significant weight loss without changes in diet or exercise may be a sign of cancer, including lung cancer.

Early detection of respiratory cancer can significantly improve the chances of successful treatment. Do not ignore these symptoms, as early intervention can make a significant difference in managing the disease.

Skin Symptoms

Skin symptoms refer to changes and abnormalities in the skin that may signal the presence of a malignant tumor or skin cancer. They vary depending on the type of skin cancer or other cancers that may manifest on the skin, but here are some common signs to watch out for:

- **New or Changing Moles:** The sudden appearance of new moles or changes such as size, shape, color, or irregular borders of existing moles may be a sign of melanoma, an aggressive type of skin cancer.

- **Non-healing Skin Lesions:** Skin wounds or ulcers that do not heal or that recur frequently may be a sign of skin cancer, especially squamous cell carcinoma.

- **Unusual Skin Rashes:** Persistent skin rashes, itching, or unexplained redness of the skin may be related to various types of cancer, including cutaneous lymphoma and basal cell carcinoma.

- **Chronic Itching:** Intense and persistent itching of the skin, especially when accompanied by other skin symptoms, should be evaluated by a healthcare professional.

- **Skin Changes Around the Nipples:** Skin changes around the nipples, such as the appearance of crusts, scales, or ulcers, may be associated with breast cancer.

- **Redness or Swelling of the Skin:** Persistent redness of the skin, especially on the chest, may be a sign of inflammatory breast cancer.

- **White Spots or Skin Discoloration:** White spots or areas of skin discoloration that cannot be explained by other dermatological causes should be examined.

- **Swollen Lymph Nodes:** The presence of swollen lymph nodes in the affected skin area may indicate that cancer has spread to other parts of the body.

Unusual skin changes should not be ignored. Consult a dermatologist or doctor if you notice any of these symptoms, as early diagnosis can be crucial for the treatment and effective management of skin cancer or other skin cancers.

Urinary Symptoms

Urinary symptoms refer to abnormalities or changes in the urinary system that may be associated with the presence of a malignant tumor in organs such as the bladder, kidneys, prostate, or urinary tract. They can vary depending on the type of cancer and its location, but here are some common signs to consider:

- **Blood in the Urine (Hematuria):** The presence of visible blood in the urine, whether red or pink, is a concerning symptom that may be related to various types of cancer, including bladder cancer, kidney cancer, or prostate cancer.

- **Pain or Burning During Urination:** Pain or burning during urination may be the result of a urinary tract infection, but it can also be associated with bladder or prostate cancer.

- **Frequent Urination:** A significant increase in the frequency of urination, especially at night, may be a symptom of prostate or bladder cancer.

- **Difficulty Urinating:** Difficulty starting urination, a weak urinary stream, or a sensation of incomplete bladder emptying may be signs of prostate cancer or urinary obstruction.

- **Urgent Urination Needs:** A sudden and strong urge to urinate that cannot be delayed may be a symptom of bladder cancer.

- **Abdominal Swelling or Pain in the Lower Back:** Unexplained abdominal swelling or pain in the lower back may be associated with kidney cancer.

- **Frequent Urinary Tract Infections:** Recurrent urinary tract infections, especially in men, may be a sign of prostate cancer.

- **Unexplained Weight Loss:** Significant weight loss without changes in diet or exercise may be a sign of cancer, including certain types of kidney cancer.

These symptoms may also be attributed to other health problems unrelated to cancer, such as urinary tract infections or urological disorders. However, anyone experiencing any of these signs should consult a healthcare professional for an accurate diagnosis.

Gynecological Symptoms

Gynecological symptoms can indicate the presence of malignant tumors in female reproductive organs, including the breasts, uterus, ovaries, cervix, or vulva. Here are some common signs to consider:

- **Breast Changes:** Any changes in breast size, shape, or texture, or the appearance of lumps, nodules, pain, redness, or unusual nipple discharge, may be signs of breast cancer.

- **Pelvic or Abdominal Pain:** Persistent, unexplained pelvic or abdominal pain unrelated to the menstrual cycle may be associated with ovarian or uterine cancer.

- **Abnormal Menstruation:** Abnormal menstruation, including heavy, prolonged, irregular, or intermenstrual bleeding, may be a sign of uterine or cervical cancer.

- **Pain During Sexual Intercourse:** Dyspareunia, or pain during sexual intercourse, may be related to vulvar, vaginal, or cervical cancer.

- **Changes in Vaginal Discharge:** Abnormal vaginal discharge, such as foul-smelling discharge, discharge with blood, or unusual color, may be signs of gynecological cancer.

- **Abdominal Swelling:** Unexplained abdominal swelling or a sensation of abdominal distension may be associated with ovarian or uterine cancer.

- **Urinary or Bowel Disorders:** Frequent urinary problems such as frequent or painful urination, as well as bowel disorders such as persistent constipation, may be symptoms of advanced gynecological cancers pressing on neighboring organs.

- **Unexplained Weight Loss**: Significant weight loss without changes in diet or exercise may be a sign of advanced gynecological cancer.

- **Lower Back or Leg Pain:** Persistent lower back or leg pain, especially if associated with other gynecological symptoms, may be a sign of advanced gynecological cancer.

Early detection of gynecological cancers is crucial for effective treatment, so it is imperative not to ignore these warning signs and to seek medical evaluation if there are concerns.

Oral Symptoms

Oral symptoms can indicate the presence of malignant tumors in the oral cavity, including the mouth, tongue, gums, cheeks, palate, or throat. Here are some common signs and symptoms associated with oral cancer:

- **Oral Ulcers:** Mouth ulcers or lesions that do not heal within a reasonable timeframe may be a sign of oral cancer. These ulcers can be painful and persistent.

- **Unusual Sores or Lesions:** The appearance of sores, lesions, nodules, or crusts in the mouth or on the lips, especially if they have irregular edges or bleed easily, should be examined by a healthcare professional.

- **Changes in Color or Texture of Oral Tissues:** Changes in the color or texture of oral tissues, such as red, white, or rough areas, may indicate a potential problem, including oral cancer.

- **Persistent Oral Pain:** Persistent oral pain, which may radiate to the ear or throat, may be associated with oral or throat cancer.

- **Difficulty Chewing or Swallowing:** If you experience difficulty chewing, swallowing, or moving the tongue, it may be a symptom of oral or throat cancer.

- **Swelling of Neck Lymph Nodes:** Swelling of neck lymph nodes may indicate that cancer has spread to the lymph nodes, which is common in the case of oral cancer.

- **Persistent Bad Breath:** Persistent bad breath that does not improve despite good oral hygiene may be related to an oral problem or oral cancer.

- **Unexplained Weight Loss:** Significant weight loss without changes in diet or exercise may be a sign of oral cancer, especially in the advanced stages of the disease.

- **Numbness or Loss of Sensation:** Numbness or loss of sensation in the mouth, tongue, or lips may be a concerning symptom.

- **Changes in Voice:** Changes in voice, such as persistent hoarseness or raspiness, may be associated with throat or oral cancer.

It is essential not to ignore these warning signs and to seek medical evaluation if there are concerns. Regular visits to the dentist and self-examination of the oral cavity can also help spot potential symptoms at an early stage.

General Symptoms

General symptoms related to cancer are bodily or physiological signs that may manifest as malignant disease progresses in the body. It is important to note that these symptoms are not specific to cancer, meaning they can be associated with many other medical conditions. However, it is crucial to consider any persistent or unexplained symptom and consult a healthcare professional for proper evaluation. Here are some of the general symptoms commonly associated with cancer:

- **Persistent Fatigue:** Extreme and persistent fatigue that does not improve with rest can be a sign of cancer. It may be due to the increased energy demand of the body to fight the disease or anemia caused by certain cancers.

- **Unexplained Weight Loss:** Significant weight loss without changes in diet or exercise can be a concerning symptom. It may be related to decreased appetite due to cancer, increased energy consumption by the tumor, or loss of muscle mass.

- **Unexplained Fever:** Persistent fever without an apparent cause can be a symptom of certain types of cancer, including lymphoma and leukemia, as abnormal production of blood cells can disrupt the immune system.

- **Excessive Night Sweats:** Frequent and excessive night sweats, particularly when accompanied by fever, may be associated with certain cancers, including lymphoma.

- **Anorexia:** Loss of appetite and disinterest in food can be early signs of certain digestive cancers or side effects of cancer itself or its treatments.

- **Changes in Lymph Nodes:** Swelling or tenderness of the lymph nodes, especially if painless, can be a sign of cancer, as it may indicate that cancer has spread to the lymph nodes.

- **Chronic Pain:** Persistent and unusual pain in a part of the body may be related to tumor growth and is often a symptom of cancer.

- **Changes in Skin:** Skin changes such as the appearance of spots, nodules, or unexplained skin lesions can be warning signs, especially if accompanied by itching, bleeding, or changes in color.

- **Changes in Bowel or Urinary Habits:** Changes in bowel or urinary habits, such as color, consistency, or the presence of blood, should be reported to a healthcare professional as they may indicate digestive or urological cancer.

- **Hormonal Changes:** Abnormal hormonal changes may be associated with certain types of cancer, such as breast cancer or thyroid cancer.

In conclusion, it is essential to consult a healthcare professional if you experience persistent symptoms, even if they seem benign. Never ignore unexplained changes in your health and always seek medical advice when necessary.

The Importance of Early Detection

Early cancer screening is the process by which healthcare professionals look for signs of the disease in individuals who show no apparent symptoms. The importance of early cancer screening cannot be overstated as it plays a crucial role in the prevention, detection, and effective treatment of this devastating illness.

Here are some reasons why early cancer screening is so crucial:

- Improved chances of recovery: In many cases, when cancer is diagnosed at an early stage, the chances of recovery are significantly higher. Malignant tumors detected early are generally smaller and less likely to have spread to other parts of the body, making them more accessible to treatment.

- **Reduction of morbidity and mortality:** Early screening helps detect cancers before they cause severe symptoms or major complications. This can reduce morbidity (negative impact on quality of life) and mortality (death) related to cancer.

- **Less invasive treatments:** When cancer is detected early, it's often possible to opt for less invasive treatments such as minimally invasive surgery, targeted radiotherapy, or gentler drug therapies. This can reduce side effects and improve patients' quality of life.

- **Cost savings:** Early cancer detection can reduce treatment costs by avoiding more aggressive and prolonged treatments, as well as by reducing costly hospitalizations and palliative care.

- **Prevention of metastasis:** Early screening can help prevent or minimize the spread of cancer to other organs, which can significantly increase long-term survival chances.

- **Awareness and education:** Early screening programs also raise awareness among the population about the importance of healthy lifestyles, self-examination, and regular medical care-seeking. This can contribute to an overall reduction in cancer risk.

- **Continuous monitoring:** For individuals at increased risk of cancer due to factors such as family history, regular screening can enable continuous monitoring and early detection of any abnormalities.

- **Opportunity to participate in clinical trials:** Patients whose cancer is diagnosed at an early stage sometimes have the opportunity to participate in clinical trials for new treatments and experimental therapies, which can offer advanced treatment options.

It's important to note that early screening doesn't just involve specific cancers but also screening strategies that vary based on age, gender, and individual risk factors. It's essential to discuss with a healthcare professional to determine appropriate screening recommendations based on your personal profile.

Cancer Treatments

Treatment Options

Cancer treatment relies on various therapeutic options, which are selected based on the type of cancer, its stage, the patient's overall health, and other individual factors. The main cancer treatment options include:

- **Surgery:** Surgery is often the primary option to remove the malignant tumor from the body. It can be used to remove part or all of the tumor, as well as nearby lymph nodes that may be affected. Surgery can be curative when the tumor is localized, or it can be used in conjunction with other treatments such as chemotherapy or radiation therapy.

- **Chemotherapy:** Chemotherapy involves using anticancer drugs to destroy cancer cells or slow their growth. These drugs can be administered intravenously or orally and can target cancer throughout the body. Chemotherapy is often used for cancers that have spread to other parts of the body (metastases) or to prevent their recurrence after surgery.

- **Radiation therapy:** Radiation therapy involves using ionizing radiation to destroy cancer cells or reduce their size. It is often used to treat solid tumors, such as breast, lung, and prostate cancers. Radiation therapy can be delivered externally (from a machine) or internally (radioactive implants).

- **Immunotherapy:** Immunotherapy boosts the patient's immune system to help fight cancer. It uses specific drugs that target cancer cells or modify the immune system to recognize and attack them. Immunotherapy has revolutionized the treatment of certain types of cancer, such as lung cancer and melanoma.

- **Targeted therapy:** Targeted therapy uses drugs that are designed to specifically target genetic or molecular abnormalities present in cancer cells. It can be used for cancers that have specific mutations, such as HER2-positive breast cancer or KRAS-mutant colon cancer.

- **Hormone therapy:** Hormone therapy is used for cancers that are influenced by hormones, such as breast or prostate cancer. It involves blocking or suppressing hormone production or blocking their action on cancer cells.

- **Gene therapy:** Gene therapy is an innovative approach that genetically modifies the patient's immune cells to make them more effective in fighting cancer. It is still in development and is primarily used in clinical trials.

- **Palliative care:** Palliative care aims to improve the quality of life for cancer patients by managing symptoms, providing psychological support, and helping patients cope with the emotional aspects of the disease. It is not aimed at curing cancer but at relieving pain and improving well-being.

Often, a multidisciplinary approach is used, where multiple treatment modalities are combined to maximize effectiveness while minimizing side effects. It is essential to discuss the available treatment options in detail with your medical team and to actively participate in decision-making to find the best strategy for your particular case.

Side Effects

Cancer treatments are essential for fighting the disease, but they can lead to various side effects. These effects vary depending on the treatment, individual sensitivity, and patient tolerance. It is important to understand that each person reacts differently to treatments, and some may experience milder side effects than others. Here is a more detailed description of common side effects associated with cancer treatments:

Chemotherapy

- Nausea and vomiting: These symptoms are common during and after a chemotherapy session, but anti-nausea medications can help alleviate them.

- Fatigue: Chemotherapy can cause extreme fatigue that can last for several days or weeks.

- Hair loss: Some types of chemotherapy result in temporary hair loss.

- Decreased red blood cell count (anemia): This can cause increased fatigue and shortness of breath.

- Decreased white blood cell count (neutropenia): This makes the patient more vulnerable to infections.

- Decreased platelet count (thrombocytopenia): This can cause excessive bleeding or easy bruising.

Radiotherapy

- Skin irritation: The skin in the treated area may become red, dry, and irritated.

- Fatigue: Radiation therapy can lead to increased fatigue, especially when administered over a long period.

- Gastrointestinal problems: Issues such as diarrhea or difficulty swallowing may occur if the radiation therapy targets the abdominal region or throat.

- Urinary problems: Pelvic radiation therapy may increase urinary frequency or cause burning during urination.

Immunotherapy

- Skin reactions: Rashes, itching, or redness may occur.

- Fatigue: Fatigue may be a side effect of immunotherapy.

- Autoimmune reactions: Immunotherapy can trigger autoimmune reactions, where the immune system attacks healthy tissues.

Targeted Therapy

- Hypertension: Some targeted therapies may increase blood pressure.

- Heart problems: They may also increase the risk of heart problems.

Hormone Therapy

- Hot flashes: Women undergoing hormone therapy may experience hot flashes similar to those of menopause.

- Bone density loss: Long-term hormone therapies may increase the risk of bone density loss (osteoporosis).

- Emotional effects: Cancer treatment can have emotional repercussions, including anxiety, depression, and sleep disturbances.

There are often ways to mitigate side effects. Healthcare professionals may recommend medications, supportive therapies, or other strategies to help patients. Therefore, it is essential to maintain open communication with your doctor and nurses throughout treatment to ensure the best possible quality of life during this challenging time.

Long-Term Effects

Some cancer treatments can lead to long-term risks, meaning that side effects or treatment-related complications may occur well after the completion of the initial treatment. Here are some examples:

- **Chemotherapy Drug Toxicity:** Some chemotherapies can damage healthy cells in the body in addition to cancer cells, leading to long-term side effects. For example, this may include heart problems, fertility issues, peripheral neuropathies (nerve damage), or increased risks of developing other cancers.

- **Radiation Therapy Side Effects:** Radiation therapy can damage healthy tissues surrounding the area targeted by the treatment. This can result in long-term issues such as fibrosis (hardening of tissues), heart problems, lung problems, or an increased risk of developing other cancers in the irradiated area.

- **Immunosuppression:** Some treatments, such as chemotherapy, can weaken the patient's immune system, making them more vulnerable to infections. This may persist even after the end of treatment, exposing the patient to an increased risk of long-term infections.

- **Mental Health Issues:** The diagnosis of cancer and its treatment can have a significant psychological impact. Patients may face mental health issues such as depression, anxiety, and post-traumatic stress, which may persist long-term.

It is essential to note that long-term risks vary depending on the type of cancer, stage of the disease, specific treatments, and the individual patient's response. The choice of treatment will always depend on a thorough assessment of benefits and risks, and patients should be thoroughly informed about the short-term and long-term implications of their treatment plan. Thus, open communication with the medical team is essential for informed decision-making and optimal risk management.

Prevention and Recurrence

The Importance of Prevention in Cancer

The old saying *"Prevention is better than cure"* makes perfect sense when it comes to dealing with cancer. Instead of relying on treatment after diagnosis, investing in preventive measures can make all the difference.

- **Risk Reduction:** By adopting a healthy lifestyle, avoiding known risk factors, and undergoing regular screening, the chances of developing cancer can be significantly reduced.

- **Cost Savings:** Cancer treatment can be financially burdensome for individuals and healthcare systems. Prevention saves not only money but also valuable medical resources.

- **Quality of Life:** Avoiding cancer often means avoiding difficult treatments and the accompanying side effects. This translates to a better quality of life for individuals and their loved ones.

- **Longevity:** Cancer prevention can contribute to a longer and healthier life. By adopting healthy lifestyle habits, one can hope to live longer without being affected by this disease.

Prevention and Screening

The distinction between primary prevention and secondary prevention is essential to understand the comprehensive approach to combating cancer. These two categories aim to reduce the burden of cancer, but they focus on different aspects of the disease and use distinct methods.

Primary Prevention

Primary prevention is one of the most effective approaches to reducing the incidence of cancer. It aims to prevent cancer from developing in the first place by adopting preventive measures before the first cancer cells appear. Here are some key elements of primary prevention:

- **Promotion of healthy lifestyles:** Adopting a healthy lifestyle is at the core of primary prevention. This includes balanced nutrition, regular physical activity, limiting alcohol consumption, and quitting smoking. These healthy lifestyle choices help maintain a healthy body weight and reduce cancer-related risk factors.

- **Vaccination:** Some viral infections, such as human papillomavirus (HPV), hepatitis B and C, are associated with an increased risk of developing certain types of cancer. Vaccination against these infections can significantly reduce the associated cancer risk.

- **Reduction of exposure to modifiable risk factors:** Avoiding exposure to risk factors such as excessive sun exposure without protection and carcinogenic chemicals is crucial for primary prevention.

Secondary Prevention

Secondary prevention focuses on the early detection of cancer in individuals at high risk. It aims to identify the disease at an early stage when the chances of cure are highest. Here's how secondary prevention works:

- **Regular Screening:** Medical exams are the cornerstone of secondary prevention. These tests are tailored based on the type of cancer and individual risk factors. For example, mammograms are commonly used for early detection of breast cancer in women, while colonoscopies are used for colon cancer.

- **Medical Surveillance:** Individuals considered at high risk due to their family history, genetic predispositions, or other factors may undergo closer medical surveillance. This may include more frequent exams or more sensitive screening tests.

Secondary prevention is particularly crucial for cancers that can have a silent progression without apparent symptoms in the early stages of development. Early screening allows for action to be taken before the disease progresses and becomes more challenging to treat.

Preventing Cancer Recurrence

Cancer recurrence is an important topic to address when discussing this disease. After receiving treatment for cancer and being in remission, there is always a risk of the cancer coming back. This is known as cancer recurrence, and it is a crucial aspect of battling this disease.

Cancer Recurrence Statistics

Cancer recurrence statistics vary significantly depending on the type of cancer, the stage at the time of diagnosis, the treatment received, and other individual factors. Here are some general statistics regarding cancer recurrence for certain common types:

- **Breast Cancer:** Recurrence rates for breast cancer vary depending on the stage at the time of diagnosis. For example, the 5-year recurrence rate for early stages is generally around 5 to 10%, while for advanced stages, it can reach 30% or more. The risk of breast cancer recurrence may persist for many years after initial treatment, and it may increase over time, especially in women with hormone-dependent breast cancer.

- **Lung Cancer:** Lung cancer tends to have a higher recurrence rate, especially in people with advanced stages at the time of diagnosis. 5-year recurrence rates can range from 40% to over 80% depending on the stage and type of cancer.

- **Colorectal Cancer:** The recurrence rate for colorectal cancer depends on the stage at the time of diagnosis and the complete removal of tumors during surgery. The 5-year recurrence rate for early stages is generally around 10%, while for more advanced stages, it can reach 30% or more.

- **Prostate Cancer:** Prostate cancer typically has a slower recurrence rate. For patients with early-stage prostate cancer who have undergone radical prostatectomy, the 5-year recurrence rate is generally around 10%.

- **Cervical Cancer:** The recurrence rate of cervical cancer depends on the stage at the time of diagnosis and the response to treatment. Recurrence rates vary, but for advanced stages, they can be higher.

- **Skin Cancer (Melanoma):** Melanoma recurrence rates depend on the stage at the time of diagnosis. For early stages, the 5-year recurrence rate is around 10%, while for advanced stages, it can be much higher.

It is essential to note that these statistics are general and may not necessarily reflect the individual situation of each patient. Additionally, new cancer treatments and management approaches are continually being developed, which may influence recurrence rates. For accurate information on cancer recurrence, it is recommended to consult an oncologist specialized in treating your type of cancer and discuss your personal situation in detail.

Risk Factors for Recurrence

Several factors can influence the risk of cancer recurrence. These factors include:

- **Cancer Type:** Some types of cancer have a higher risk of recurrence than others. For example, breast cancer and prostate cancer tend to have a relatively high risk of recurrence.

- **Cancer Stage:** The stage at the time of initial diagnosis is a determining factor. Cancers diagnosed at a more advanced stage often have a higher risk of recurrence.

- **Initial Treatment:** The type of initial treatment received can also influence the risk of recurrence. Some treatments are more effective than others in preventing recurrence.

- **Personal Risk Factors:** Personal risk factors such as smoking, excessive alcohol consumption, obesity, and exposure to carcinogens can increase the risk of recurrence.

Managing Recurrence

It is important to note that cancer recurrence is not necessarily a death sentence. Many patients with recurrence can benefit from additional treatments or targeted therapies to manage the disease. Regular monitoring and follow-up examinations are essential for quickly detecting any recurrence and intervening promptly.

Medical Research

Investing in medical research is a fundamental pillar in the fight against cancer, and its importance cannot be overstated. The significant progress made in understanding the disease and developing more effective treatments is the result of decades of dedicated research.

Medical research has allowed us to better understand the underlying mechanisms of cancer. This includes understanding the genetic mutations that lead to the formation of cancer cells, as well as the complex biological processes that promote their growth and spread. This in-depth knowledge has paved the way for more targeted and personalized treatment approaches.

Moreover, many cancer treatments have been developed, ranging from surgery and radiotherapy to targeted therapies and immunotherapy. These advancements have significantly improved survival rates and the quality of life for cancer patients. Targeted treatments specifically aim at cancer cells, thereby reducing undesirable side effects. Research also continues to explore new therapeutic approaches for cancer treatment. This includes identifying new molecular targets, developing innovative drugs, researching immunotherapy, and utilizing gene therapy to specifically target cancer cells. These advancements pave the way for more effective and less invasive treatments.

Investment in research also aims to prevent the disease at an early stage. Epidemiological and genetic studies help identify cancer risk factors, which can guide prevention programs. Additionally, research contributes to the development of more sensitive and specific screening tests, allowing for the detection of cancer at an increasingly early stage when chances of cure are highest.

It also aims to make treatments more accessible. This includes research on less expensive treatments, the development of generic drugs, and reducing financial barriers for patients. The goal is to ensure that the most advanced treatments are available to all who need them, regardless of their economic situation.

Cancer research is often conducted internationally, with collaboration between scientists, researchers, and clinicians from around the world. This collaboration promotes the rapid dissemination of knowledge, the exchange of ideas, and the establishment of multicenter clinical trials, accelerating the development of new therapeutic approaches.

It is important to recognize that cancer research also faces challenges. Clinical trials can be lengthy and costly, and not all treatments under development prove to be effective. However, every advance in understanding cancer and developing new therapies represents a step forward in the fight against this disease.

Conclusion

Throughout this chapter, we have explored different types of cancer, examined alarming global statistics, discussed risk factors and symptoms, and emphasized the crucial importance of early detection. We have also touched on available treatments and highlighted the importance of managing side effects.

Cancer may seem daunting, but it is important to remember that knowledge is our most powerful ally in this battle. By understanding cancer from all angles, we can better arm ourselves to fight it.

Now that we have a solid foundation, it is time to examine the link between diet and cancer. Therefore, in the next chapter, we will discover how the choices we make at every meal can play a crucial role in cancer prevention and management.

Nutrition and Cancer

Introduction

Over the decades, scientific research has illuminated the complex pathways through which our diet influences our cells, metabolism, and ultimately, our health. In this chapter, we will explore how certain foods can promote or suppress cell growth, how inflammation and oxidation can play a decisive role, and how the choices we make on our plate can have lasting consequences on our well-being. We will also discover how organic food can influence our health, and we will separate myths from realities so that you can make informed decisions about nutrition.

The Link Between Diet and Cancer

Diet is a key element of our overall well-being and quality of life, but it is also a powerful double-edged sword: it can protect us against many diseases, including cancer, but also increase our vulnerability to these conditions.

Therefore, it is essential to understand how our diet can affect our health in order to make informed dietary choices for long-term health and to adopt a proactive approach in reducing the risks of developing serious illnesses. Rather than relying on expensive and potentially taxing medical treatments once the disease has set in, prevention offers us a safer and more economical path to living a healthy and productive life.

Furthermore, our health influences every aspect of our lives, from our relationships to our ability to work and enjoy the activities we love. Understanding how our diet can improve our quality of life by reducing the risk of cancer and other diseases encourages us to make wiser dietary choices. By investing in a healthy diet, we can hope to live a longer, more active, and more fulfilling life.

Ultimately, by understanding the impact of our diet on our health, we can also set an example for future generations. Our eating habits are often passed down to our children and grandchildren. By making informed dietary choices, we can help create a healthier food environment for future generations.

Underlying Mechanisms

Cellular Promotion and Suppression

Diet plays a crucial role in regulating cellular promotion and suppression, significantly impacting the risk of cancer development. Understanding how certain foods and nutrients influence these processes can help adopt a diet that promotes cellular health and reduces the risk of cancer.

Cellular Promotion

Cellular promotion refers to the stimulation of cell growth and division, including cancer cells. Some foods and dietary habits can promote cellular promotion and increase the risk of cancer. Here's how diet can influence this process:

- **Foods high in empty calories:** Excessive consumption of foods high in empty calories, such as sugary drinks, highly processed snacks, and foods high in sugar and saturated fat, can lead to excessive weight gain. Obesity is a major risk factor for cancer because fat cells produce hormones and inflammatory cytokines that promote abnormal cell growth.

- **Diets rich in processed meats:** Diets rich in processed meats, such as deli meats and processed red meats, have been associated with an increased risk of certain cancers, including colorectal cancer. Chemicals and compounds present in these foods can damage the DNA of cells and promote tumor growth.

- **Excessive alcohol consumption:** Excessive alcohol consumption is a well-established risk factor for several types of cancer, including breast, liver, esophageal, and oral cancer. Alcohol can directly damage the DNA of cells and disrupt DNA repair mechanisms.

- **Foods high in saturated fats:** Saturated fats found in animal-based foods and processed foods can trigger chronic inflammation in the body, thus promoting cellular promotion and tumor growth.

Cellular Suppression

Cellular Suppression, on the other hand, involves preventing the growth and uncontrolled proliferation of cells, including cancer cells. Some dietary compounds can have cellular suppression properties and help reduce the risk of cancer. Here's how diet can influence this process:

- **Antioxidants:** Antioxidants found in fruits, vegetables, and legumes, such as vitamins C and E, beta-carotene, and polyphenols, help protect cells against oxidative damage by neutralizing free radicals. They play a crucial role in cellular suppression by reducing the risk of genetic mutations and DNA damage that could lead to cancer.

- **Dietary Fiber:** Foods rich in dietary fiber, such as whole grains, vegetables, and fruits, are associated with a reduced risk of cancer, especially colon cancer. Dietary fiber can contribute to cellular suppression by promoting intestinal regularity and eliminating potentially harmful toxins from the intestinal tract.

- **Isoflavones and Phytoestrogens:** These compounds found in legumes and soy-based products may have cellular suppression properties by mimicking the effects of female hormones and reducing the risk of certain hormone-dependent cancers, such as breast and prostate cancer.

- **Glucosinolates:** Cruciferous vegetables, such as broccoli, cauliflower, and Brussels sprouts, contain compounds called glucosinolates, which have been associated with a reduced risk of cancer. These compounds can stimulate cellular suppression mechanisms and help eliminate precancerous cells.

Inflammation and Oxidative Stress

In order to understand how chronic inflammation and oxidative stress are linked to cancer development, it is essential to delve into the complex world of cellular biology. These two processes play a crucial role in the context of the disease, and their understanding can help prevent and fight cancer more effectively.

Chronic Inflammation

Inflammation is a natural response of the body to injury or infection. However, when this inflammation becomes chronic, it can become problematic. When immune cells are constantly activated due to persistent inflammation, they can damage healthy tissues and promote the development of cancerous cells. Some chronic inflammatory diseases, such as ulcerative colitis, are also linked to an increased risk of cancer.

Oxidative Stress

Oxidative stress is a process that occurs when the body produces an excess of free radicals, unstable molecules that damage cells. This stress can be caused by various factors, including an unhealthy diet, smoking, exposure to toxins, and even psychological stress. When cells are exposed to oxidative stress for prolonged periods, they undergo DNA damage, which can potentially trigger genetic mutations leading to cancer.

Complex Links with Cancer

Chronic inflammation and oxidative stress are not independent processes. In reality, they are closely linked. Chronic inflammation can contribute to oxidative stress by activating immune cells that produce free radicals. In turn, free radicals can trigger inflammation. This complex interaction creates an environment conducive to cancer development.

Prevention Strategies

Fortunately, there are ways to control chronic inflammation and oxidative stress. A diet rich in antioxidants, such as vitamins C and E, as well as regular physical activity, can reduce oxidative stress. Managing mental stress, through relaxation and meditation techniques, can also help reduce chronic inflammation. By adopting a healthy lifestyle, everyone can contribute to minimizing these cancer risk factors.

Hormonal Impact

When discussing the influence of diet on cancer, it is essential to understand the crucial role of hormones, especially in women. Indeed, hormones such as estrogen and progesterone are essential for many normal bodily functions, including the regulation of the menstrual cycle, fertility, and pregnancy. However, high levels of sex hormones, particularly in women, have been associated with an increased risk of cancer. This includes types of cancer such as breast, uterine, and ovarian cancer.

Dietary Influences on Hormones

Diet plays a fundamental role in hormone regulation. Some foods can help balance hormone levels, while others can disrupt them. For example, a diet rich in fiber from fruits, vegetables, and whole grains can help eliminate excess hormones from the body. On the other hand, excessive consumption of processed foods rich in saturated fats can contribute to hormonal imbalances.

The Role of Phytoestrogens

Phytoestrogens, found in certain plant-based foods, are compounds that resemble the body's natural estrogens. They can bind to estrogen receptors and influence hormone levels.

For example, isoflavones found in soy are phytoestrogens that may have beneficial effects on hormonal health.

Omega-3s and Antioxidants

Omega-3 fatty acids, found in fatty fish such as salmon, as well as antioxidants found in berries and cruciferous vegetables, have shown positive effects on hormonal regulation and reducing the risk of cancer in women.

The Role of Organic Diet

The role of organic diet in cancer prevention is garnering increasing interest as more people turn to organic foods to promote their health. While research in this field is ongoing, some studies suggest that organic foods may have a positive impact on reducing the risk of cancer.

Reduced Pesticide Residues

One of the primary reasons people choose organic foods is the reduction of pesticide residues. Organic crops are grown without the use of synthetic chemical pesticides. This means that organic fruits, vegetables, grains, and other organic products are less likely to contain potentially harmful pesticide residues. Studies have shown that long-term exposure to pesticides may be associated with an increased risk of certain types of cancer, including breast cancer and prostate cancer.

Absence of GMOs

Organic foods typically exclude genetically modified organisms (GMOs). While the safety of GMOs for human consumption is debated, and more research is needed to establish a clear link, there are concerns about the potential effects of GMOs on health, including their link to certain types of cancer, and many people choose to avoid GMOs.

More Nutrients and Antioxidants

Some proponents of organic diet claim that organic foods may contain more nutrients and antioxidants than conventional foods. This may be due to farming practices that promote soil and plant health, resulting in better nutritional quality. Antioxidants, abundant in many organic fruits and vegetables, can help reduce oxidative stress, which is linked to cancer development.

Fewer Food Additives

Organic foods tend to contain fewer food additives, such as colorings, preservatives, and artificial flavors. Some food additives have been associated with health issues, and avoiding excessive consumption of them could have a positive impact on reducing the risk of cancer.

Overall Healthier Diet

People who adopt an organic diet tend to be more health-conscious and make overall healthier food choices. They often have a greater propensity to consume fresh foods, vegetables, fruits, organic dairy products, and meats from organically raised animals. This can contribute to an overall healthier diet, which is an important factor in cancer prevention.

Myths vs. Facts

When it comes to cancer, many misconceptions circulate, often fueled by popular beliefs or misleading information that spreads quickly. In this section, we will debunk these common myths and present scientifically validated information on the relationship between diet and cancer to enable you to make informed decisions regarding diet and cancer prevention.

Sugar Does Not Feed Cancer

The myth: One of the most widespread myths is that sugar fuels cancer growth. It is true that cancer cells have a voracious appetite for glucose (sugar), but this does not mean that consuming sugar necessarily makes cancer grow. In reality, all cells in our body, including healthy cells, need glucose to function. The key is to maintain a balance.

The facts: Completely avoiding sugar is neither necessary nor recommended. However, it is wise to limit the consumption of added sugars found in sodas, candies, and pastries. Instead, opt for sources of complex carbohydrates such as whole grains, vegetables, and fruits.

Antioxidants Do Not Cure Cancer

The myth: Antioxidants, found in foods like fruits, vegetables, and dietary supplements, are often touted for their cancer-fighting properties. While they play a crucial role in protecting our cells against oxidative damage, the idea that antioxidants cure cancer is simplistic.

The facts: Antioxidants are not a miracle cure for cancer. Their main role is to prevent cellular damage that could promote cancer development. Studies have shown that high levels of certain antioxidants may interfere with the effectiveness of chemotherapy. It is best to obtain antioxidants from a balanced diet rather than taking them in supplement form.

Coffee Does Not Cause Cancer

The myth: Coffee is one of the most consumed beverages worldwide, and it has often been associated with an increased risk of cancer, especially bladder cancer. This association has raised concerns and misunderstandings.

The facts: Several studies have examined the relationship between coffee consumption and cancer risk. Overall, research shows that moderate coffee consumption does not appear to increase the risk of cancer. In fact, coffee contains bioactive compounds, such as polyphenols and antioxidants, that could have protective effects against certain types of cancer. However, moderation is essential, as excessive coffee consumption can have other adverse effects on health.

Organic Foods Do Not Prevent Cancer

The myth: Organic foods are becoming increasingly popular as they are perceived as healthier and free from pesticides. Some even believe they can prevent cancer.

The facts: Organic foods may have benefits in terms of reducing pesticide exposure, but there is no solid evidence that they specifically prevent cancer. Overall dietary choices, such as consuming fruits, vegetables, whole grains, and lean proteins, have a greater impact on cancer prevention than simply opting for organic foods.

Keto or Low-Carb Diets Are Not the Key to Prevention

The myth: Keto (ketogenic) and low-carb diets have become popular for weight loss and are sometimes touted as miracle solutions for preventing cancer by starving cancer cells of glucose.

The facts: Keto diets may be effective for weight management, but their use for cancer prevention is debatable. Some studies suggest they might be helpful in cancer treatment, but research is ongoing. A balanced diet rich in fiber, vegetables, fruits, and lean proteins is generally recommended for cancer prevention, rather than sticking to extremely restrictive diets.

Not All Dairy Products Promote Cancer

The myth: Some people believe that all dairy products, especially milk, increase the risk of cancer due to their hormone and saturated fat content.

The facts: Studies on dairy products and cancer are mixed. The link between dairy products and cancer depends on the type of cancer and the amount of dairy consumed. Dairy products can be an important source of calcium and vitamin D, which may have protective effects against certain types of cancer when consumed in moderation.

Spicy Foods Do Not Cause Stomach CancerTop of Form

The myth: There is a belief that spicy foods, such as chili peppers, can irritate the stomach lining and increase the risk of stomach cancer.

The facts: Spicy foods themselves are not associated with stomach cancer. However, a diet high in heavily salted or smoked foods may increase the risk of stomach cancer. Spices can be consumed in moderation as part of a balanced diet.

Raw Foods Are Not Always Better Than Cooked Foods

The myth: Some believe that primarily eating raw foods is healthier because cooking would destroy nutrients.

The facts: Cooking can indeed reduce the content of certain nutrients, but it can also make other nutrients more bioavailable. For example, cooking vegetables can destroy enzymes responsible for digesting fiber, thus facilitating their absorption. It is important to maintain a balance between raw and cooked foods to benefit from all nutrients.

Late-night Eating Does Not Promote Cancer

The myth: Some believe that eating late at night leads to weight gain and increases the risk of cancer.

The facts: When you eat is less important than what you eat and how much you consume. Total calories and the quality of your diet have a greater impact on your weight and health than the time you eat. However, eating too close to bedtime can disrupt your sleep, which can have a negative impact on your long-term health.

Gluten-Free Products Are Not Better for Cancer Prevention

The myth: Some believe that gluten-free diets, increasingly popular, are better for cancer prevention.

The facts: Gluten-free diets are essential for people with celiac disease or gluten sensitivity, but there is no solid evidence that gluten-free diets specifically prevent cancer in non-gluten-sensitive individuals. Cancer prevention depends more on a balanced diet rich in fiber, weight management, and a healthy lifestyle in general.

Conclusion

In this chapter dedicated to the link between diet and cancer, we have discussed underlying mechanisms, debunked common myths, and highlighted the importance of making informed dietary choices.

We understand that diet can be a powerful tool in our overall health and in cancer prevention. By making wise dietary choices and adopting a healthy diet, we can contribute to strengthening our resilience against this formidable disease.

Now that we have explored this solid foundation, we are prepared to delve deeper into the world of foods, nutrients, and anti-cancer dietary supplements in the next chapter. We will explore current knowledge and practical strategies for effective anti-cancer nutrition.

The Warriors of the Plate

Introduction

In our exploration of anticancer nutrition, we now embark on a journey to discover the true heroes of your plate: the foods that are powerful allies in the fight against cancer.

These superfoods, as we call them, are much more than mere ingredients in our diet. They are nutritional gems rich in essential nutrients, antioxidants, vitamins, minerals, and phytochemical compounds. Their potential in cancer prevention and management is considerable.

We will also delve into the world of dietary supplements, nutritional reinforcements that can help bridge the gaps in our daily diet, highlighting their potential benefits in the fight against cancer while emphasizing the importance of using them safely and effectively.

Furthermore, we will not forget to discuss the foods we should avoid or limit. Processed foods, high in saturated fats and additives, as well as excessive sugars, are not our allies in this battle. We will discuss the dangers they pose and strategies to avoid them.

This chapter aims to arm you with practical knowledge about the foods that can be valuable assets in your anticancer arsenal. You will learn to choose wisely what you put on your plate to maximize nutritional benefits and strengthen your defense against cancer.

Superfoods

Introduction to Superfoods

Definition of Superfoods

Superfoods, as the name suggests, are foods distinguished by their exceptional nutritional density. They are typically rich in essential nutrients such as vitamins, minerals, antioxidants, dietary fibers, and healthy fats. What characterizes superfoods is their ability to provide a high concentration of these beneficial nutrients per serving, making them outstanding choices for health.

Superfoods often come from nature, whether they are fruits, vegetables, seeds, nuts, berries, or other plant-based products. However, some animal products, such as wild salmon, are also considered superfoods due to their high content of omega-3 fatty acids and other beneficial nutrients.

What particularly distinguishes superfoods is their ability to provide health benefits beyond basic nutrition. They are often associated with medicinal properties, disease prevention, and overall well-being promotion. These exceptional foods have become popular due to their ability to support general health and reduce the risk of many conditions, including cancer.

Superfoods in Anti-Cancer Nutrition

Superfoods play a key role in anti-cancer nutrition due to their specific properties that contribute to the prevention and management of this dreaded disease. Here's why superfoods are essential in cancer prevention and management:

- **Antioxidants and Reduction of Oxidative Stress:** Superfoods are often rich in antioxidants, such as vitamins C and E, selenium, polyphenols, and carotenoids. These compounds neutralize free radicals and reduce oxidative stress, which can damage cells and contribute to cancer development.

- **Natural Anti-Inflammatories:** Many superfoods have natural anti-inflammatory properties. Chronic inflammation is linked to an increased risk of cancer, and regular consumption of superfoods can help reduce inflammation in the body.

- **DNA Protection:** Some superfoods contain compounds that help protect DNA from damage and genetic mutations. This can reduce the risk of cellular transformation that leads to cancer.

- **Detoxification:** Some superfoods, such as kale, Brussels sprouts, and broccoli, promote the body's natural detoxification by helping the liver eliminate harmful substances. Effective detoxification can help eliminate potential carcinogens.

- **Immune System Boost:** Superfoods often stimulate the immune system by providing vitamins, minerals, and other essential nutrients that support immune functions. A strong immune system is essential for detecting and eliminating cancer cells.

- **Anti-Angiogenic Effects:** Some superfoods have anti-angiogenic effects, meaning they inhibit the formation of new blood vessels nourishing tumors. This can slow down tumor growth.

Key Nutrients in Superfoods

Antioxidants

Antioxidants are compounds found abundantly in many superfoods, and they play a crucial role in cancer prevention and overall health preservation. Here's how antioxidants work and why they are essential:

- **Function of Antioxidants:** Free radicals are unstable molecules naturally produced by cellular metabolism and exposed to environmental factors such as pollution, tobacco, and UV rays. These free radicals can damage cells and DNA, thereby contributing to cancer development. Antioxidants work by neutralizing these free radicals, rendering them harmless.

- **Prevention of Cellular Damage:** Cellular damage caused by free radicals can lead to genetic mutations, inflammation, and cellular transformation processes. Antioxidants help prevent this damage by inhibiting the oxidation of cellular components.

- **Importance in Cancer Prevention:** Numerous epidemiological studies have shown that regular consumption of foods rich in antioxidants, such as berries, citrus fruits, nuts, and leafy green vegetables, is associated with a reduced risk of cancer. Antioxidants help protect cells against mutations that could make them cancerous.

Here are some examples of antioxidants and the foods in which they are found:

- Vitamin C: Found in citrus fruits (such as oranges, lemons, and grapefruits), strawberries, kiwis, red bell peppers, and spinach.

- Vitamin E: Present in nuts, seeds, wheat germ oil, olive oil, and avocados.

- Beta-carotene: Found in carrots, sweet potatoes, spinach, squash, mangoes, and apricots.

- Selenium: Present in Brazil nuts, sunflower seeds, fish, turkey, and eggs.

- Flavonoids: Found in berries (such as blueberries and raspberries), green tea, apples, red onions, and dark chocolate.

- Zinc: Found in shellfish (such as oysters), beef, chicken, legumes, and nuts.

- Resveratrol: Present in red wine, red grapes, berries, and peanuts.

- Lutein and zeaxanthin: Found in leafy green vegetables (such as spinach and kale), eggs, and corn.

- Polyphenols: Present in tea, coffee, red fruits, leafy green vegetables, and red wine.

- Coenzyme Q10 (CoQ10): Found in fatty fish (such as salmon and tuna), nuts, liver, and soy.

These antioxidants help protect the body's cells and tissues from oxidative damage and play a role in promoting overall health. It is important to include a variety of antioxidant-rich foods in a balanced diet to maximize their health benefits.

Phytonutrients

Phytonutrients, also known as phytochemicals, are bioactive substances naturally found in plants. They give fruits, vegetables, herbs, and spices their distinctive colors, flavors, and medicinal properties. Phytonutrients are crucial in cancer prevention for the following reasons:

- Cancer Protection: Many phytonutrients have demonstrated anticancer properties, including the ability to inhibit the growth of cancer cells, induce their programmed death (apoptosis), and block the formation of new blood vessels to tumors (angiogenesis).

- Immune System Support: Some phytonutrients, such as carotenoids (like beta-carotene), flavonoids, and glucosinolates, strengthen the immune system by helping regulate immune functions. A robust immune system is essential for detecting and destroying cancer cells.

- Reduction of Inflammation: Many phytonutrients have anti-inflammatory properties. They help reduce chronic inflammation, which is a major risk factor for cancer. For example, anthocyanins found in berries have powerful anti-inflammatory effects.

- Diversity and Variety: Phytonutrients are found in a wide variety of foods. Therefore, it is essential to consume a variety of superfoods to benefit from a wide range of phytonutrients. Carrots (rich in beta-carotene), spinach (rich in lutein), and green tea (rich in catechins) are some examples of foods rich in phytonutrients.

Here are some examples of phytonutrients and the foods in which they are found:

- Flavonoids: Present in citrus fruits (such as oranges and lemons), berries (such as blueberries and strawberries), leafy green vegetables (such as spinach and broccoli), and tea, flavonoids have antioxidant and anti-inflammatory properties.

- Carotenoids: Found in carrots, sweet potatoes, spinach, mangoes, and bell peppers. Carotenoids such as beta-carotene are converted into vitamin A in the body, which is essential for eye and skin health.

- Glucosinolates: Present in cruciferous vegetables such as broccoli, cauliflower, kale, and radishes, glucosinolates can help detoxify the body and have potential anticancer properties.

- Polyphenols: Found in red wine, green tea, dark chocolate, red fruits, and vegetables like onions and shallots. Polyphenols are known for their antioxidant and anti-inflammatory properties.

- Quercetin: Present in apples, onions, citrus fruits, and tea, quercetin is a flavonoid that can contribute to cardiovascular health and reduce inflammation.

- Curcumin: Found in turmeric, a yellow spice often used in Indian cuisine, curcumin has powerful anti-inflammatory and antioxidant properties.

- Lignans: Present in flaxseeds, sesame seeds, and whole grains, lignans have beneficial effects on heart and hormonal health.

- Phytosterols: Found in nuts, seeds, leafy green vegetables, and vegetable oils, phytosterols can help reduce blood cholesterol levels.

These phytonutrients are an essential component of a healthy and balanced diet and can offer a variety of health benefits when regularly included in the diet.

Vitamins and Minerals

Superaliments are often rich in vitamins and minerals, which are essential micronutrients for many biological functions in the body. Here are some examples of vitamins and minerals commonly found in superaliments and their roles in health:

- Vitamin C: Found in citrus fruits, berries, peppers, and broccoli, vitamin C boosts the immune system, promotes wound healing, and acts as an antioxidant.

- Vitamin E: Found in nuts, seeds, and olive oil, vitamin E protects cells against oxidative damage and strengthens the immune system.

- Vitamin D: Found in fatty fish (such as salmon) and mushrooms, vitamin D is essential for bone health and immune function.

- Selenium: Selenium, found in Brazil nuts, fish, and eggs, is a mineral that acts as an antioxidant and helps protect DNA in cells.

- Zinc: Zinc, found in pumpkin seeds, lentils, and lean meat, is essential for cell growth, wound healing, and immune function.

- Calcium: Found in dairy products and leafy green vegetables, calcium is essential for bone health and cell regulation.

List of Anticancer Superfoods

Plant-Based Superfoods

Plant-based superfoods are an essential component of an anticancer diet. They are rich in beneficial nutrients, antioxidants, and phytonutrients. Here are some examples of plant-based superfoods and how they contribute to cancer prevention:

Fruits and Vegetables

- Berries: Berries, such as strawberries, blueberries, and raspberries, are rich in antioxidants, particularly vitamin C and polyphenols, which help reduce the risk of cancer by neutralizing free radicals.

- Broccoli and Cauliflower: These cruciferous vegetables contain sulfur compounds, such as glucosinolates, which have anticancer properties by promoting detoxification and suppressing abnormal cell growth.

- Spinach and Kale: Rich in lutein, vitamin K, and fiber, these green vegetables help reduce the risk of cancer by supporting cellular health and reducing inflammation.

Whole Grains

- Oats: Oats are rich in soluble fiber, which helps maintain healthy bowel regularity, reducing the risk of colorectal cancer.

- Quinoa: This grain is a valuable source of plant-based protein, fiber, and many nutrients, contributing to a balanced diet that supports overall health.

Legumes

- Lentils: Lentils are rich in fiber, plant-based protein, and folate, which play a role in DNA repair, helping to prevent genetic mutations.

Unique Foods

- Turmeric: This spice contains curcumin, a compound with anti-inflammatory and antioxidant properties. Turmeric is linked to reducing the risk of cancer, especially colorectal cancer.

- Raw Honey: Raw honey is rich in antioxidants and has antimicrobial properties. It can support overall health by boosting the immune system.

Sea Vegetables

- Spirulina and Chlorella: These algae are rich in protein, chlorophyll, and essential nutrients. They can support the immune system and promote detoxification.

Superfoods of Animal Origin

While most superfoods are derived from plants, there are certain animal-based products that are also considered beneficial for health and may contribute to cancer prevention. Here are some examples of animal-based superfoods and their advantages:

Fatty Fish

- Wild Salmon: Wild salmon stands out as an excellent source of omega-3 fatty acids, such as eicosapentaenoic acid (EPA) and docosahexaenoic acid (DHA), which possess anti-inflammatory properties and are associated with a reduced risk of cancer, particularly breast cancer.

Dairy Products

- Active Cultured Yogurt: Yogurts containing probiotic cultures promote intestinal health by fostering a balanced gut microbiome. A healthy digestive system is correlated with a lowered risk of colon cancer.

Eggs

- Omega-3 Enriched Eggs: Eggs fortified with omega-3 fatty acids offer a rich source of high-quality protein and essential fats, contributing to a well-rounded diet and potentially aiding in cancer prevention.

It's worth noting that while animal-based superfoods offer health benefits, moderation is key, and it's advisable to prioritize a diet primarily composed of plant-based sources to optimize health benefits and mitigate the risk of cancer.

Practical Tips

- Prioritize fresh and unprocessed foods: Fresh and unprocessed foods, such as fruits, vegetables, whole grains, lean meats, and unprocessed dairy products, are rich in essential nutrients. They provide vitamins, minerals, antioxidants, and dietary fiber that are important for health. By choosing these foods, you ensure better nutritional quality in your diet. Processed foods, on the other hand, are often high in added sugars, saturated fats, and additives that can be detrimental to health.

- Avoid overcooking, which can degrade nutrients: Overcooking food, especially cooking at high temperatures, can lead to the loss of essential nutrients. Some vitamins, like vitamin C, are sensitive to heat and can be destroyed with excessive cooking. Vegetables can also lose their nutrients if they are overcooked. To preserve the maximum nutrients, it is recommended to steam, quickly stir-fry, or eat foods raw whenever possible. Avoiding overcooking helps maintain the nutritional value of foods.

- Drink enough water throughout the day: Water is essential for many bodily functions, including digestion, waste elimination, regulation of body temperature, and nutrient transport. Adequate hydration is important for maintaining your overall health. When you are well-hydrated, it can also help control your appetite and maintain your energy levels. It is recommended to drink about 8 glasses of water per day, but water needs can vary depending on your age, weight, activity level, and environmental conditions. Staying hydrated is essential for optimal anticancer nutrition.

Summary Table

Here is a summary table of the leading anticancer foods and their key beneficial nutrients:

Anticancer Foods	Key Nutrients
Broccoli	Indole-3-carbinol, vitamin C, fiber
Kale	Antioxidants (carotenoids, flavonoids), vitamin K, fiber
Spinach	Folate, vitamin K, iron, antioxidants (lutein, zeaxanthin)
Turmeric	Curcumin (powerful antioxidant)
Tomatoes	Lycopene, vitamin C, potassium, folate
Garlic	Allicin, sulfur compounds, antioxidants
Green Tea	Catechins, polyphenols
Blueberries	Anthocyanins, vitamin C, fiber
Flaxseeds	Omega-3 fatty acids, lignans, fiber
Walnuts	Omega-3 fatty acids, antioxidants, fiber

Warnings and Limits of Superfoods

While superfoods offer an impressive range of nutrients and health benefits, it is essential not to focus exclusively on them at the expense of a balanced and diversified diet. Here's why maintaining dietary balance is important:

- Nutrient Complementarity: Although exceptional, superfoods cannot provide all the nutrients the body needs in sufficient quantities. A balanced diet includes a variety of food sources to ensure adequate intake of proteins, carbohydrates, fats, vitamins, and minerals.

- Caloric Balance: Some superfoods, such as nuts and avocados, are calorically dense. Consumed in excess, they can contribute to excessive calorie intake, which can lead to unwanted weight gain.

- Nutritional Diversity: Dietary diversity ensures that one benefits from the widest range of nutrients possible. Each food has its own benefits and specific nutrients, and superfoods do not cover all nutritional needs.

- Enjoyment of Food: Food is more than just a source of nutrients. It is also a source of pleasure and conviviality. Restricting oneself only to superfoods can make the diet monotonous and less satisfying taste-wise.

In summary, it is important to consider superfoods as a beneficial component of your diet, but they should not monopolize your eating habits. For overall balanced and anticancer nutrition, it is best to integrate them into a varied dietary framework that includes a wide range of foods from both plant and animal sources.

Zooming in on Supplements

Introduction to Dietary Supplements

Definition of Dietary Supplements

Dietary supplements are substances taken in addition to regular food to supplement the intake of essential nutrients. They can come in the form of pills, capsules, powders, liquids, gels, or tablets. Dietary supplements contain a variety of nutrients, including vitamins, minerals, amino acids, fatty acids, enzymes, herbs, plant extracts, and other bioactive compounds.

In the context of anticancer nutrition, dietary supplements are relevant because they can help fill nutritional gaps, boost the immune system, reduce inflammation, and provide specific nutrients that support cancer prevention and treatment. They are generally used alongside a balanced diet and healthy lifestyle to maximize health benefits.

Amplification of Superfoods Effects

Dietary supplements can play an important role in amplifying the effects of superfoods in cancer prevention and treatment. Here's how supplements can work synergistically with superfoods:

- Supplementation of Essential Nutrients: Sometimes, it can be challenging to obtain sufficient amounts of certain nutrients from diet alone. Supplements can fill these nutritional gaps by providing essential vitamins and minerals. For example, vitamin D, which can be synthesized by the body through sunlight exposure, can also be taken as a supplement to maintain adequate levels, which can be important in cancer prevention.

- Boosting the Immune System: Some supplements can support the immune system, which is crucial for detecting and destroying cancer cells.

- Additional Antioxidants: While many superfoods are rich in antioxidants, taking supplements containing specific antioxidants such as vitamin C, vitamin E, or selenium can help strengthen the body's ability to neutralize free radicals and reduce oxidative stress.

- Plant-Based Supplements: Some dietary supplements contain extracts of medicinal plants, such as turmeric, green tea, or resveratrol, which have anti-inflammatory and anticancer properties.

- Adaptogens: Some dietary supplements, such as ashwagandha or ginseng, are considered adaptogens. They help the body adapt to stress and can support overall health, which is essential for cancer prevention.

Star Anticancer Supplements

Star anticancer dietary supplements are supplements that have stood out in research and clinical practice for their potential to support cancer prevention and treatment. They are often chosen for their anti-inflammatory, antioxidant, immunomodulatory, and other mechanisms that may contribute to reducing the risk of cancer. Here are some of these star dietary supplements and their potential benefits:

- Curcumin: Curcumin is the active compound in turmeric, a spice widely used in Asian cuisine. It is recognized for its anti-inflammatory, antioxidant, and anticancer properties. Curcumin can help reduce chronic inflammation, inhibit the growth of cancer cells, and promote programmed cell death (apoptosis).

- Quercetin: Quercetin is a flavonoid found in many fruits, vegetables, and teas. It has demonstrated potential anticancer effects by suppressing the growth of cancer cells, inhibiting the formation of blood vessels in tumors (angiogenesis), and stimulating the immune system.

- Resveratrol: Resveratrol is a polyphenol found in red grapes, red wine, and certain pome fruits. It has antioxidant and anti-inflammatory properties. Resveratrol is studied for its potential role in reducing the risk of cancer, especially breast cancer and prostate cancer.

- Selenium: Selenium is an essential mineral found in many foods, including Brazil nuts, fish, meat, and eggs. It is a key component of antioxidant enzymes and can help protect cells against oxidative damage. Studies have shown that adequate levels of selenium are associated with a reduced risk of certain types of cancer, such as prostate cancer.

- Vitamin D: Vitamin D is essential for bone health, but it also plays a role in regulating cell growth and the immune system. Adequate levels of vitamin D are associated with a reduced risk of certain cancers, including colorectal cancer, breast cancer, and prostate cancer.

- Omega-3: Omega-3 fatty acids, found in fatty fish like salmon and fish oil supplements, have anti-inflammatory properties. They can reduce chronic inflammation, which is a risk factor for many types of cancer.

Safe and Effective Use of Supplements

Dosage and Frequency

The use of dietary supplements for anticancer nutrition should be approached with caution and by following the recommended doses. Here are some guidelines on the quantity and frequency of supplement use, focusing on safety:

- Adhere to Recommended Dosages: It is essential to follow the instructions on the supplement label regarding the recommended daily dose. Overconsumption of certain nutrients can be harmful to health.

- Balance with Diet: Dietary supplements should not replace a balanced and varied diet. They are intended to complement the diet, not replace it. Superfoods and fresh foods should remain the primary source of nutrients.

- Synergy with Superfoods: When taking supplements in combination with superfoods, make sure not to exceed the overall recommended doses of nutrients. For example, if you are taking a vitamin D supplement in addition to eating salmon, make sure not to exceed the total recommended daily dose of vitamin D.

Medical Consultation

Before starting to take dietary supplements, especially in the context of anticancer nutrition, it is imperative to consult a healthcare professional. Here's why medical consultation is essential:

- Assessment of Individual Needs: A healthcare professional can assess your specific nutritional needs based on your health status, medical history, current diet, and any ongoing medical treatments. Each person has unique nutritional needs, and a personalized approach is essential to maximize benefits while minimizing risks.

- Avoiding Drug Interactions: Some dietary supplements may interact with medications you are already taking. A healthcare professional can alert you to these potential interactions and recommend safer alternatives if necessary.

- Monitoring Side Effects: Although most dietary supplements are safe when taken according to recommended doses, side effects may occur. A healthcare professional can monitor your response to supplements and adjust the dose if necessary.

In conclusion, dietary supplements can be a valuable asset in enhancing the beneficial effects of superfoods, but they should be used thoughtfully. The safe and effective use of dietary supplements in the context of anticancer nutrition relies on adhering to recommended doses, seeking medical consultation beforehand, and customizing the approach based on individual needs.

FAQs on Supplements

Q1: What are the most effective dietary supplements for cancer prevention?

There is no single supplement that guarantees cancer prevention. However, some supplements such as vitamin D, curcumin, omega-3 fatty acids, resveratrol, and selenium have shown potential anticancer effects. The key is to use them appropriately and in addition to a balanced diet.

Q2: Can I get all the nutrients I need from my diet?

Ideally, the majority of your nutrients should come from your diet. However, in some situations, supplements may be necessary to fill nutritional gaps or enhance cancer prevention. Consult a healthcare professional to assess your specific needs.

Q3: Are dietary supplements safe?

Most dietary supplements are safe when taken according to recommended doses. However, side effects may occur, especially at excessive doses. It is essential to follow instructions and consult a healthcare professional to avoid potential risks.

Q4: Can I take multiple supplements at the same time?

Yes, you can take multiple supplements at the same time, but it should be done thoughtfully. Ensure you do not exceed the total recommended doses of nutrients, and consider consulting a healthcare professional for a personalized approach.

Q5: Can dietary supplements replace a healthy diet?

No, dietary supplements should not replace a healthy and varied diet. They are meant to complement the diet, not replace it. Superfoods, fruits, vegetables, whole grains, lean proteins, and other fresh foods remain essential for optimal anticancer nutrition.

Q6: Can I take dietary supplements if I am currently undergoing cancer treatment?

If you are undergoing cancer treatment, it is essential to consult your oncologist or a healthcare professional before taking dietary supplements. Some supplements may interact with ongoing medical treatments, necessitating medical supervision.

Q7: When during the day should I take my dietary supplements?

Most dietary supplements can be taken with meals for better absorption. However, always follow the specific instructions on the supplement label, as recommendations may vary depending on the type of supplement.

Q8: How long does it take to see results with anticancer dietary supplements?

Results vary from person to person, and it may take several weeks or months to observe significant effects. Consistency in taking supplements and a healthy diet are essential to maximize benefits.

Q9: What dietary supplements should I avoid in the context of anticancer nutrition?

Avoid dietary supplements containing excessive doses of nutrients, be cautious of unregulated products, and be wary of supplements claiming to cure cancer. Always consult a healthcare professional for specific recommendations.

Q10: Are dietary supplements recommended for everyone in cancer prevention?

No, the need for dietary supplements varies based on age, gender, health status, and diet. Supplements are recommended only when nutritional gaps are identified or when potential benefits in cancer prevention are determined by a healthcare professional. A personalized approach is essential.

Foods to Avoid or Limit

It is important to note that cancer prevention is not just about consuming healthy foods but also involves reducing exposure to foods that may be harmful.

When discussing avoiding or limiting certain foods in the context of anticancer nutrition, it means taking steps to reduce the consumption of certain food products that are associated with an increased risk of developing cancer. It is important to understand that this does not necessarily mean a complete ban on these foods but rather a significant reduction in their presence in your daily diet.

Limiting these foods aims to minimize exposure to known risk factors, such as potential carcinogens or harmful compounds for health. This helps create a nutritional balance favorable to cancer prevention while maintaining a varied and enjoyable diet.

Processed and Unhealthy Foods

Processed Foods

Processed foods are food products that have been altered from their natural form for preservation, taste, or convenience reasons. These modifications may include the addition of sugars, trans fats, and food additives. Here is a list of common processed foods and why they should be limited in the context of anticancer nutrition:

- Sugary Drinks: Soft drinks, industrial fruit juices, and energy drinks often contain excessive amounts of added sugar, which can contribute to obesity, a risk factor for several types of cancer.

- Salty and Sweet Snacks: Chips, cookies, cakes, and other processed snacks are often high in trans fats, sugar, and salt. They are associated with inflammation and an increased risk of certain cancers.

- Processed Grain Products: Sweetened breakfast cereals, granola bars, and industrial bakery products are often loaded with added sugars. They can cause spikes in blood sugar levels and promote inflammation.

- Prepared Meals: Ready meals, frozen dishes, and fast food are often high in saturated fats, sodium, and additives. Excessive consumption of these foods can contribute to obesity and health problems associated with cancer.

- Processed Sauces and Condiments: Pasta sauces, condiments, and commercial dressings often contain added sugars, salt, and additives. They can make meals more calorie-dense and less healthy.

The reason for limiting these processed foods lies in their ability to increase the risk of cancer by promoting inflammation, contributing to obesity, causing spikes in blood sugar, and exposing the body to harmful substances such as trans fats and food additives.

Processed Meats and Red Meats

Processed meats such as sausages, bacon, hot dogs, and deli meats are associated with an increased risk of certain types of cancer, particularly colorectal cancer. These meats typically undergo processing that may include salting, smoking, fermenting, or the addition of preservatives. These processes can produce harmful compounds such as heterocyclic amines and polycyclic aromatic hydrocarbons, which can damage DNA and promote the growth of cancer cells.

Red meats, such as beef, pork, and lamb, are also associated with an increased risk of cancer, especially colorectal cancer and prostate cancer. Excessive consumption of red meats is linked to the formation of harmful compounds during high-temperature cooking, such as heterocyclic amines and polycyclic aromatic hydrocarbons.

In the context of anticancer nutrition, it is recommended to limit the consumption of processed meats and red meats. Opting for alternatives such as poultry, fish, vegetables, legumes, and plant-based protein sources can help reduce the cancer risk associated with these foods.

The Dangers of Saturated and Trans Fats

Saturated Fats

Saturated fats are fatty acids found in large quantities in certain animal-based foods and in some processed products. Here is a discussion on the sources of saturated fats and their potential impact on cancer:

- Sources of Saturated Fats: The main sources of saturated fats include high-fat dairy products (butter, cheese, cream), fatty meats (beef, pork), poultry skin, coconut oil, and palm oil.

- Potential Impact on Cancer: Saturated fats are associated with chronic inflammation and excessive weight gain, two risk factors for cancer. Additionally, a diet high in saturated fats may increase the production of sex hormones, which can promote the growth of certain types of cancer, such as breast cancer and prostate cancer. Therefore, it is recommended to limit the consumption of saturated fats by opting for healthier alternatives, such as unsaturated fats found in nuts, avocados, and vegetable oils.

Trans Fats

Trans fats are artificial fatty acids created through a manufacturing process called hydrogenation, often used in the food industry to make vegetable oils solid at room temperature. Trans fats are particularly dangerous to health and should be avoided at all costs. Here's why:

- Sources of Trans Fats: Trans fats are typically found in processed foods such as cookies, cakes, pastries, frozen fries, solid margarines, and many fast foods. They are also naturally present in small amounts in some meats and dairy products.

- Health Impact: Trans fats are associated with an increased risk of heart disease, obesity, type 2 diabetes, and certain types of cancer. They have the ability to raise LDL cholesterol levels (the "bad" cholesterol) and lower HDL cholesterol levels (the "good" cholesterol), promoting the buildup of plaque in arteries.

- Ban or Restriction: In many countries, artificial trans fats have been banned or strictly regulated due to their harmful health effects. However, it is still essential to carefully read labels on processed foods to check for trans fat content. Opting for unprocessed foods and cooking at home with healthy oils can help avoid these dangerous fats.

In summary, both saturated and trans fats pose a health risk, including the risk of cancer. Therefore, it is important to limit their consumption by opting for a diet rich in healthy fats and avoiding processed foods high in saturated and artificial trans fats.

Excess of Sugars and Additives

Added Sugars

Added sugars are sugars that are incorporated into foods and beverages during their preparation or processing. They differ from sugars naturally present in foods such as fruits and dairy products. Overconsumption of added sugars is a major issue in many societies, and it poses health risks, including the risk of cancer. Here's why it's important to limit added sugars in anticancer nutrition:

- Sources of Added Sugars: The main sources of added sugars include sweetened beverages (sodas, sweetened fruit juices), desserts (cakes, cookies, ice cream), candies, sweetened breakfast cereals, sauces, and condiments (ketchup, barbecue sauce).

- Health Impact: Overconsumption of added sugars can contribute to obesity, chronic inflammation, increased risk of type 2 diabetes, and promotion of cancer cell growth. Cancer cells also feed on glucose, a type of sugar, underscoring the importance of maintaining stable blood sugar levels.

- Tips: To limit added sugars, it's recommended to prioritize a diet based on fresh, unprocessed foods. When purchasing packaged products, read labels carefully to identify hidden sugars under names such as high-fructose corn syrup, sucrose, dextrose, or maltose. Opt for natural sweeteners such as raw honey or maple syrup in moderate amounts.

Food Additives

Food additives are substances added to foods for various reasons, such as preservation, coloring, texture, or flavor. Some food additives are considered safe, while others pose potential health risks. In the context of anticancer nutrition, it's important to understand these risks and know how to avoid them:

- Potential Risks: Some food additives, such as artificial colorings, artificial sweeteners (like aspartame), preservatives (like sodium nitrate), and emulsifiers, have raised concerns about their impact on health. They can contribute to inflammation, disrupt the balance of gut flora, and increase the risk of certain types of cancer.

- Reading Labels: To avoid undesirable food additives, read food product labels carefully. Additives are typically listed by their name or their E number. Learn to recognize controversial additives and prioritize unprocessed or homemade foods.

In conclusion, limiting added sugars and exercising caution regarding food additives are important practices in anticancer nutrition. Whenever possible, prioritize a diet based on fresh and natural foods that are less likely to contain potentially harmful substances.

Strategies to Avoid These Foods

Transitioning to a Healthier Diet

Transitioning to a healthier diet, which limits the consumption of foods to avoid or limit in the context of anticancer nutrition, can be a beneficial change for health. Here are some practical tips to help you make this transition smoothly:

- Make Healthy Substitutions: Identify the foods to avoid or limit in your current diet and find healthier alternatives. For example, replace sugary sodas with sparkling water with a slice of lemon, or opt for vegetable snacks instead of chips.

- Plan Your Meals: Develop a weekly meal plan that incorporates healthy and varied foods. This will help you avoid turning to processed foods for convenience.

- Cook at Home: Prepare as many meals as possible at home, where you have better control over the ingredients you use. Cooking at home helps avoid unwanted additives and fats.

- Read Labels: When grocery shopping, read food product labels carefully to spot added sugars, saturated fats, and additives. Choose products with a short and recognizable ingredient list.

- Explore New Foods: Be open to trying new foods and discovering healthy alternatives. Fruits, vegetables, legumes, whole grains, and lean proteins are excellent options.

The Importance of Moderation

It is essential to understand that moderation is key in anticancer nutrition. While some foods may be associated with an increased risk of cancer, it does not mean they should be completely eliminated from your diet. Here's why moderation is important:

- Preserve the Pleasure of Eating: Completely eliminating certain foods can make eating less enjoyable and sustainable. By allowing occasional indulgences, you maintain the pleasure of eating and avoid strict diets in the long run.

- Balance Your Diet: Moderation allows you to maintain balance in your diet. You can occasionally enjoy a dessert or processed dish while promoting an overall healthy diet.

- Reduce Food Stress: Overly restrictive diets can lead to food-related stress. By being able to manage your diet moderately, you reduce stress related to food choices.

- Overall Prevention: Cancer prevention depends not only on the elimination of specific foods but also on an overall healthy diet, physical exercise, and other lifestyle factors. Moderation helps you maintain overall balance.

In summary, transitioning to a healthier diet and practicing moderation are important strategies to avoid risky foods in anticancer nutrition. These approaches promote a sustainable, balanced, and beneficial diet for cancer prevention.

Conclusion

In this chapter, we have explored the world of superfoods and dietary supplements that can become powerful allies in the prevention and fight against cancer. You have discovered how to judiciously integrate these elements into your daily diet to strengthen your anticancer arsenal.

One of the crucial lessons from this chapter is that by choosing the right foods and understanding their impact on your health, you have the power to actively contribute to your well-being.

In the next chapter, we will delve into the realm of anticancer diets. We will continue to guide you through updated information and practical strategies for effective anticancer nutrition.

The Anticancer Diets

Introduction

Diet plays a significant role in our health, and dietary regimes can be valuable tools in our fight against cancer. Over the years, many dietary approaches have emerged, each with its own characteristics and specific benefits.

In this chapter, we will delve deep into dietary regimes designed to support cancer prevention and treatment. We will examine key diets, highlighting their potential advantages as well as any potential drawbacks. Our goal is to provide you with the necessary information to choose the diet that best suits your needs and lifestyle.

To facilitate understanding of the differences and similarities between these diets, we will use comparative tables. Whether you are drawn to the Mediterranean diet, veganism, the ketogenic diet, or other dietary approaches, we will guide you in selecting the diet that best fits you.

Key Anticancer Diets

Introduction to Dietary Regimes

An anticancer diet is a specific dietary approach designed to help prevent and fight cancer. This type of diet is based on selecting foods and nutrients that are associated with cancer-protective properties. The primary goal of an anticancer diet is to reduce dietary risk factors while promoting a diet rich in beneficial nutrients for health.

The concept of a diet rests on the idea that what we eat can influence our risk of developing cancer. By adopting a diet specifically formulated to reduce inflammation, support the immune system, and provide protective antioxidants and phytonutrients, one can potentially reduce the risk of cancer and improve response to treatments.

The choice of diet is crucial in cancer prevention and treatment. Here's why it's essential to select the right dietary regime:

- Influence on Cancer Risk: Scientific studies have shown that diet can play a significant role in the development of certain types of cancer. An anticancer diet can help reduce dietary risk factors, such as the consumption of saturated fats, added sugars, and processed foods.

- Support for Treatment: For people with cancer, a tailored diet can provide essential nutrients needed to maintain strength and vitality during treatments such as chemotherapy and radiotherapy. It can also help manage side effects such as weight loss and nausea.

- Promoting Remission: After cancer treatment, a proper diet can support remission and healing. It can help strengthen the immune system and maintain optimal health.

- Promotion of Overall Health: Even for people without cancer, an anticancer diet can contribute to overall health promotion by reducing the risk of many other chronic diseases, such as heart disease and diabetes.

The Mediterranean Diet

The Mediterranean diet is based on the eating habits of Mediterranean countries such as Greece, Italy, and Spain. It is characterized by a high consumption of:

- Extra Virgin Olive Oil: Olive oil is the main source of fat in this diet. It is rich in monounsaturated fatty acids, which are associated with a reduced risk of heart disease and certain types of cancer.

- Fruits and Vegetables: The Mediterranean diet emphasizes the consumption of fruits, vegetables, legumes, nuts, and seeds. These foods are rich in vitamins, minerals, fiber, and antioxidants.

- Fish: Fatty fish such as salmon, tuna, and sardines are regularly consumed. They provide omega-3 fatty acids, beneficial for heart health and inflammation reduction.

- Whole Grains: Whole grains, such as whole wheat and barley, are preferred over refined grains.

- Moderate Red Wine: Red wine is often consumed in moderation, which is associated with beneficial effects on heart health, although excessive alcohol consumption is discouraged.

The Mediterranean diet is associated with many health benefits, including a reduced risk of heart disease, type 2 diabetes, and certain types of cancer. It is rich in antioxidants, dietary fiber, and healthy fats, making it a solid choice in cancer prevention.

The Vegetarian / Vegan Diet

Vegetarian and vegan diets focus on the exclusion of meat, fish, and animal products (vegan). These diets mainly consist of:

- Fruits and Vegetables: A diet rich in fruits and vegetables provides an abundance of vitamins, minerals, antioxidants, and dietary fiber.

- Legumes: Legumes such as beans, lentils, and chickpeas provide plant-based protein, fiber, and essential nutrients.

- Whole Grains: Whole grains, whole wheat pasta, and brown rice are sources of complex carbohydrates and fiber.

- Nuts and Seeds: Nuts, seeds, and nut-based products provide healthy fats and protein.

- Plant-Based Products: Plant-based substitutes such as tofu and almond milk are commonly used.

Vegetarian and vegan diets are associated with a reduced risk of cancer, especially colon, breast, and prostate cancers. Their richness in antioxidants, dietary fiber, and phytonutrients can help protect cells against damage and reduce inflammation.

The Ketogenic Diet

The ketogenic diet is a very low-carbohydrate diet that promotes the production of ketones in the body, an alternative source of energy. Although it is primarily used for managing epilepsy and weight loss, it also garners interest in cancer research.

Some scientists are studying the potential of the ketogenic diet to slow down the growth of cancer cells, as they typically rely on glucose for their energy. However, more research is needed to evaluate its effectiveness and safety in cancer treatment.

The Antioxidant-Rich Diet

An antioxidant-rich diet is characterized by a high consumption of foods containing natural antioxidants, such as vitamins C and E, beta-carotene, and selenium. These antioxidants help neutralize free radicals and prevent cellular damage.

This diet includes foods such as fruits (berries, citrus fruits), vegetables (spinach, broccoli), nuts (almonds, cashews), seeds (sunflower seeds, flaxseeds), and legumes (beans, lentils).

An antioxidant-rich diet may contribute to protecting cells against damage and reducing the risk of cancer overall.

The Japanese Diet

The traditional Japanese diet is based on the eating habits of Japan. It emphasizes:

- Fatty Fish: Fatty fish, rich in omega-3 fatty acids, is an important protein source in this diet.

- Soy: Soy in various forms, including tofu and miso, is widely consumed.

- Vegetables and Seaweed: Vegetables, seaweed (such as nori), and rice are key components.

- Green Tea: Green tea is a popular beverage rich in antioxidants.

The Japanese diet is considered beneficial for health, especially regarding reducing the risk of heart disease and certain types of cancer. Foods rich in fatty fish, soy, and antioxidants contribute to its potential health benefits.

In summary, these key anticancer diets focus on specific dietary choices aimed at promoting better health. Each of these diets has its own benefits and should be tailored to individual dietary preferences. Therefore, it is important to consult with a healthcare professional or a nutritionist before significantly altering one's diet, especially in the case of cancer or underlying health issues.

Selecting a Diet

Advantages and Disadvantages

Advantages

Each anticancer diet offers specific advantages in cancer prevention by targeting different mechanisms. Here's how each of them can contribute to reducing the risk of cancer:

- Mediterranean Diet: This diet is rich in fruits, vegetables, legumes, and healthy fats, notably extra virgin olive oil. These foods provide a wide variety of antioxidants, vitamins, and minerals that help protect cells against damage and reduce inflammation, thus contributing to cancer prevention.

- Vegetarian / Vegan Diet: Vegetarian and vegan diets are naturally high in fiber, promoting healthy digestion and potentially reducing the risk of colon cancer.

Additionally, the high consumption of vegetables and fruits provides a variety of antioxidants that help combat free radicals, thus reducing the risk of cancer.

- Ketogenic Diet: Although research on the ketogenic diet's impact on cancer prevention is ongoing, this diet is being studied for its potential to starve cancer cells of glucose, forcing them to use ketones for energy. However, its effectiveness and safety remain subjects of debate, and it is generally used as a complement to traditional treatments.

- Antioxidant-Rich Diet: Antioxidants present in this diet, such as vitamins C and E, beta-carotene, and selenium, help neutralize free radicals that can damage cell DNA and promote cancer cell growth. Cancer prevention is a major benefit of this diet.

- Japanese Diet: The traditional Japanese diet is associated with a low incidence of certain types of cancer, especially breast and prostate cancer. Fatty fish rich in omega-3, soy, vegetables, and green tea are key elements of this diet, providing a variety of bioactive compounds that may contribute to cancer prevention.

Disadvantages

While each anticancer diet has advantages, it's also important to consider the potential disadvantages and limitations associated with each of them. Here are some disadvantages and precautions to consider for each diet:

- Mediterranean Diet: Although the Mediterranean diet is overall healthy, it can be calorie-rich due to the amount of olive oil used. Therefore, portion sizes should be monitored, especially if weight concerns exist. Additionally, moderate alcohol consumption should be maintained, as overconsumption can have negative health effects.

- Vegetarian / Vegan Diet: Vegetarian and vegan diets may be deficient in certain essential nutrients, such as vitamin B12, vitamin D, iron, and calcium. Careful meal planning is important to ensure all necessary nutrients are obtained. Some individuals may also require dietary supplements to address these nutritional gaps.

- Ketogenic Diet: The ketogenic diet is strict and challenging for many people to follow due to its significant carbohydrate restrictions. It can also lead to side effects such as "keto flu" during the adaptation phase. Consulting a healthcare professional is important before adopting this diet.

- Antioxidant-Rich Diet: An antioxidant-rich diet can be beneficial, but overconsumption of isolated antioxidant supplements may have undesirable effects. It's preferable to obtain antioxidants from natural foods rather than supplements, unless otherwise advised by a healthcare professional.

- Japanese Diet: Although the traditional Japanese diet is considered healthy, it's important to note that fish consumption may lead to increased exposure to certain contaminants such as mercury. Therefore, choosing low-mercury fish, such as wild salmon or sardines, and limiting consumption of predator fish is recommended.

In summary, each anticancer diet has its advantages, but also potential disadvantages. It's essential to consider these factors before adopting a specific dietary regimen. A personalized approach to nutrition is often most suitable to meet individual needs.

How to Choose the Right Diet

The choice of the anticancer diet that best suits each person depends on various factors, including dietary preferences, lifestyle, current health, and personal goals. Here are some tips to help you select the diet that suits you best:

- Consult a Healthcare Professional: Before making a decision, consult a doctor or a nutritionist. They can assess your current health status, medical history, and specific nutritional needs.

- Consider Your Dietary Preferences: Choose a diet that fits your taste preferences. If you don't like specific foods in a given diet, it may be challenging to stick to it in the long term.

- Think About Your Lifestyle: Take your lifestyle into account. For example, if you have a very busy job, a diet that requires complex preparation may not be realistic for you.

- Listen to Your Body: Pay attention to how your body reacts to a particular diet. If you feel tired, weak, or have digestive issues, it may be a sign that the current diet is not suitable for you.

- Identify Your Goals: Clearly define your goals in adopting an anticancer diet. What do you want to achieve? Reduce the risk of cancer, support ongoing treatment, manage side effects, or improve your overall health?

- Consider Customization: An anticancer diet should be tailored to your specific needs. For example, if you have nutritional deficiencies, your diet will need to be adjusted to address these gaps.

The Importance of Customization

Customization is essential to achieve the best results. Each individual is unique, with specific nutritional needs, different dietary reactions, and varied personal goals. Here's why customization is crucial:

- Nutrition Optimization: Customizing your diet means you will get the essential nutrients your body needs to function optimally. This can help you maintain your strength, energy, and immune system during the cancer fight.

- Reduction of Side Effects: Customizing the diet can help alleviate treatment side effects, such as nausea, weight loss, and fatigue.

- Adaptation to Specific Needs: Some individuals have specific nutritional needs due to medical issues or dietary concerns. A customized diet can take these needs into account.

- Sustainability: A diet tailored to your lifestyle and dietary preferences is more likely to be sustainable in the long term, which is essential for maintaining health benefits.

- Motivation: When your diet is customized to meet your goals and needs, you are more likely to stay motivated and follow the meal plan.

Comparative Tables of Diets

Here is a table summarizing the typical composition of each anticancer diet, including the types of foods allowed and restricted:

Diet	Allowed Foods	Limited Foods
Mediterranean Diet	Fruits, vegetables, whole grains, fish, nuts, extra virgin olive oil, legumes.	Red meats, processed foods high in saturated fats and added sugars.
Vegetarian / Vegan Diet	Fruits, vegetables, whole grains, legumes, nuts, seeds, plant-based proteins.	Red meats, processed meats, dairy products, eggs (for vegan diet).
Ketogenic Diet	Lean meats, fish, avocados, nuts, seeds, healthy oils, low-carb vegetables.	Grains, high-carb fruits, carb-rich foods.
Antioxidant-Rich Diet	Fruits, vegetables, nuts, seeds, herbs.	Processed foods high in added sugars.
Japanese Diet	Fish, soy, vegetables, rice, seaweed, green tea.	Processed foods high in added sugars, saturated fats.

This table summarizes the practicality and adaptability of each diet:

Diet	Adaptability	Costs
Mediterranean Diet	Relatively easy to follow for many people, compatible with various lifestyles.	Cost depends on the availability of Mediterranean products in the region.
Vegetarian / Vegan Diet	May require careful planning to address nutritional deficiencies but is adaptable to various dietary preferences.	Generally affordable, but cost will depend on the availability of vegetarian/vegan foods.
Ketogenic Diet	May be challenging to follow due to strict carbohydrate restrictions, not suitable for all lifestyles.	Costs may be high due to purchasing lean meats, nuts, and healthy oils.
Antioxidant-Rich Diet	Can be adapted to various dietary preferences, but particular attention to food quality is essential.	Generally affordable as it emphasizes natural foods, but but costs may increase if antioxidant supplements are added.
Japanese Diet	Can be adapted to many dietary preferences, but depends on the availability of Japanese products.	Generally affordable using local foods, but quality fish can be expensive.

Conclusion

In this chapter, we embarked on a thorough exploration of various dietary approaches that play a crucial role in cancer prevention and treatment. We carefully examined the primary anticancer diets, assessed their advantages and disadvantages, and provided tools to help you select the one that best suits your individual situation. By making wise dietary choices and adopting a suitable regimen, you have the power to exert a positive influence on your health and well-being.

Now, we will delve into the fascinating universe of the microbiome. This incredible community, comprised of billions of microorganisms, primarily inhabits our digestive tract. You will discover why the microbiome is our invisible ally in the fight against cancer, with its diversity and crucial role in our overall health.

The Microbiome: The Invisible Ally

Introduction

As we continue our exploration of anticancer nutrition, we now dive into an invisible yet incredibly powerful realm that resides deep within us: the microbiome. In this chapter, we will explore the crucial role that this microscopic world plays in supporting our health and contributing to the fight against cancer.

The microbiome is a complex community of bacteria, viruses, fungi, and other microorganisms that populate our digestive tract. Far more than just a collection of gut inhabitants, the microbiome closely interacts with our body and wields considerable influence over our well-being.

In this chapter, we will examine the microbiome's crucial role in promoting health and defending against cancer. You will discover how dietary diversity can nourish and strengthen your microbiome, and how a healthy microbiome can contribute to cancer prevention and support existing treatments.

We will discuss the concept of the colorful plate and how it can promote a diverse microbiome. Prebiotics and probiotics, essential allies of your microbiome, will also take center stage. You will learn how to judiciously incorporate them into your daily diet to support your well-being.

Role of the Microbiome in Health

Introduction to the Microbiome

The microbiome, also known as the microbiota, is a term used to refer to the collection of microorganisms living inside and on the surface of the human body. These microorganisms are primarily composed of bacteria but also include viruses, fungi, and other microbes. The microbiome forms a true ecological community that interacts symbiotically with our organism.

The human microbiome is present in various parts of the body, but it is particularly studied in the context of the intestine, where the concentration of microorganisms is highest. The intestinal microbiome consists of billions of bacteria that primarily reside in the large intestine.

The composition of the microbiome can vary from person to person due to various factors, including age, gender, diet, environment, exposure to antibiotics and other medications, as well as other genetic and epigenetic factors. It is unique to each individual, much like a microbiological fingerprint.

The microbiome fulfills many crucial functions for our health and well-being. Among its essential roles, we can cite:

- Food Digestion: Microorganisms in the microbiome help break down the food we consume, especially plant fibers, to extract essential nutrients.

- Synthesis of Vitamins and Nutrients: Some bacteria in the microbiome can produce essential vitamins, such as vitamin K and certain B vitamins.

- Protection Against Pathogens: A balanced microbiome acts as a protective barrier by preventing the excessive growth of potentially harmful pathogenic microorganisms.

- Regulation of the Immune System: The microbiome influences the immune system by contributing to the formation of an appropriate immune response.

- Impact on Metabolism: The microbiome can affect metabolism, including modulating nutrient absorption and participating in appetite regulation.

- Influence on Mental Health: Recent studies suggest that the microbiome can also influence the brain, which can impact mood, behavior, and even neurological conditions.

Research on the microbiome is constantly evolving, and new discoveries are made regularly. Understanding the role of the microbiome in human health has become a major research area, and it is increasingly recognized as a key player in many diseases, including cancer. By taking care of our microbiome through diet, environment, and other factors, we can improve our health and reduce the risks of certain diseases, including cancer.

The Role of the Microbiome in Cancer

The role of the microbiome in cancer research is a rapidly growing field that has revealed the crucial importance of microbiome composition and health in the development, progression, and prevention of cancer. The precise mechanisms of interaction between the microbiome and cancer are still being explored, but here are some of the main ways in which the microbiome can influence the fight against cancer:

- Protection Against Carcinogens: A healthy microbiome can act as a protective barrier against carcinogens. By producing antibacterial substances and occupying space in the intestine, beneficial bacteria in the microbiome limit the growth of pathogenic bacteria and the formation of potentially toxic compounds.

- Inflammation and Immune Response: Chronic inflammation is a well-established risk factor in cancer development. The microbiome can influence inflammation by regulating the immune response. A balanced microbiome helps maintain moderate inflammation, while dysbiosis (microbiome imbalance) can promote excessive inflammation.

- Beneficial Metabolites: Microbiome bacteria produce metabolites, such as short-chain fatty acids, that have anti-inflammatory and immunomodulatory properties. These metabolites may play a role in preventing abnormal cell proliferation.

- Interaction with the Tumor Microenvironment: Recent studies have shown that the microbiome can interact with the microenvironment around cancer cells. Microbiome bacteria can influence the response to anticancer treatments, such as immunotherapy, by modifying local conditions around the tumor.

- Drug Metabolism: The microbiome can also influence the metabolism of anticancer drugs. Some bacteria can activate or deactivate drugs, which can impact their effectiveness and toxicity.

- Hormonal Balance: Research suggests that the microbiome can influence hormone metabolism, which can impact the risk of certain hormone-related cancers, such as breast cancer and prostate cancer.

It is important to note that the microbiome is dynamic and can be influenced by factors such as diet, antibiotics, stress, and the environment. Therefore, promoting a healthy microbiome through balanced diet, probiotics and prebiotics intake, and reducing disruptive factors is an important strategy in cancer prevention.

However, it should be emphasized that the microbiome is complex, and research is ongoing to better understand its specific mechanisms in the fight against cancer. Interventions aimed at improving microbiome health are an integral part of the comprehensive approach to cancer prevention, but they should not be considered as a single solution.

Tips for a Healthy Microbiome

Dietary Diversity

The role of dietary diversity in supporting a healthy microbiome is crucial. Dietary diversity refers to the variety of foods you consume in your daily diet. When you eat a wide range of foods from different sources, you provide your microbiome with a diverse array of nutrients, fibers, phytochemicals, and other essential elements for its health.

Here's how dietary diversity promotes a healthy and balanced microbiome:

- Feeding a Greater Variety of Bacteria: Each type of food you consume provides specific nutritional substrates for different strains of bacteria in your microbiome. By diversifying your diet, you ensure that all these bacteria have enough food to thrive. A large diversity of bacteria is associated with better gut health. Greater bacterial diversity is generally associated with better resilience of the microbiome to disturbances and diseases.

- Provides a Wider Range of Nutrients: Each food group provides specific nutrients. For example, green leafy vegetables are rich in vitamins and minerals, while legumes provide fiber and protein. A diversified diet ensures that your body receives a complete range of essential nutrients.

- Encourages the Production of Beneficial Metabolites: Gut bacteria digest the foods you consume and produce metabolites, such as short-chain fatty acids, which have positive effects on colon and immune system health. A varied diet can promote the production of these beneficial metabolites.

- Reduces the Risk of Dysbiosis: Eating the same foods repetitively can lead to an imbalance in the microbiome, called dysbiosis. Dysbiosis can promote the growth of pathogenic bacteria. By diversifying your diet, you minimize this risk.

To support a healthy microbiome, it is recommended to consume a wide variety of foods from different categories, including:

- Fruits and vegetables of all colors.
- Legumes such as beans, lentils, and peas.

- Whole grains such as oats, brown rice, and quinoa.

- Lean proteins such as chicken, fish, and tofu.

- Fermented dairy products such as yogurt and kefir (if tolerated).

- Nuts, seeds, and healthy plant oils.

It is also important to vary the methods of food preparation to maximize the diversity of nutrients available. A diversified diet can not only promote microbiome health but also contribute to better overall health and cancer prevention by providing your body with the essential elements it needs to function optimally.

The Concept of Colorful Plate

The concept of the colorful plate is a visual and simple approach to eating that emphasizes the importance of consuming a wide variety of foods, especially vegetables, fruits, and protein sources, to support a healthy microbiome and promote overall health. This method highlights the diversity of colors and types of foods found on a balanced plate and is widely recommended by nutritionists and health experts.

Here's what the colorful plate means and why it's important for microbiome health:

- Variety of Colors: A colorful plate consists of a variety of bright colors from different foods. Each color is associated with specific nutrients and beneficial phytochemicals for health. For example, green vegetables are rich in vitamin K and folate, orange carrots and peppers are high in beta-carotene, and red berries are rich in antioxidants.

141

- Provision of Essential Nutrients: Each color group represents a food group that provides essential nutrients. Green vegetables are a source of fiber, vitamins, and minerals, red fruits provide antioxidants, legumes supply protein and fiber, and fatty fish contain omega-3 fatty acids.

- Support for the Microbiome: The diversity of foods on a colorful plate also means a variety of dietary fibers, prebiotics, and other compounds that nourish beneficial bacteria in the microbiome. Fiber is particularly important for microbiome health as it serves as food for gut bacteria and promotes better bacterial diversity.

- Reduction of Dysbiosis Risk: By favoring a wide variety of foods, the colorful plate can help prevent dysbiosis, which is the imbalance of the microbiome that can promote the growth of pathogenic bacteria. A varied diet offers a greater likelihood that all microbiome bacteria have enough nutritional substrates to thrive.

- Pleasure and Satisfaction: The colorful plate makes meals more visually and gustatorily appealing. This can encourage a more balanced and enjoyable diet, promoting regularity and continuity of healthy eating.

The goal of the colorful plate is to make every meal an opportunity to nourish your body with a wide variety of nutrients and promote a healthy microbiome. By incorporating a palette of colors and flavors into your daily diet, you contribute to the nutritional diversity of your microbiome, which can have a positive impact on your long-term health, including reducing the risk of cancer and other chronic diseases.

Prebiotics to Feed the Microbiome

The Role of Prebiotics

Prebiotics are non-digestible food compounds that act as a source of nourishment for the beneficial bacteria present in the intestinal microbiome. In other words, they are substances that we cannot digest ourselves but are fermented by beneficial bacteria in our colon. Prebiotics thus contribute to promoting the growth and activity of bacteria, thereby improving the overall health of our microbiome.

Prebiotics have several beneficial effects on health, including:

- Promoting the growth of beneficial bacteria: Prebiotics nourish bacteria such as bifidobacteria and lactobacilli, which are known for their positive role in digestion, immune system regulation, and production of beneficial metabolites.

- Stimulating the production of short-chain fatty acids (SCFAs): When bacteria ferment prebiotics, they produce SCFAs such as acetate, propionate, and butyrate. These SCFAs have anti-inflammatory effects and can strengthen the intestinal barrier.

- Lowering the pH of the colon: Fermentation of prebiotics by bacteria produces acids that lower the pH of the colon. This can inhibit the growth of pathogenic bacteria and promote a more favorable environment for beneficial bacteria.

- Improving mineral absorption: Prebiotics can enhance the absorption of certain minerals, such as calcium and magnesium, in the colon.

Foods Rich in Prebiotics

Prebiotics are mainly found in foods rich in dietary fiber, especially soluble fibers. Here are some examples of foods rich in prebiotics:

- Vegetables: Garlic, onions, leeks, asparagus, artichokes, and chicory are rich in fructans, a form of prebiotics.

- Fruits: Bananas, apples, pears, prunes, and berries contain prebiotics in the form of pectins.

- Legumes: Lentils, chickpeas, beans, and peas are an excellent source of prebiotics, especially fructans.

- Whole grains: Whole grains such as oats, whole wheat, and barley contain prebiotics in the form of beta-glucans and other soluble fibers.

- Fermented foods: Fermented foods such as yogurt, kefir, sauerkraut, and kimchi may also contain prebiotics, in addition to probiotic bacteria.

Incorporating these prebiotic-rich foods into your daily diet can help support the health of your microbiome by providing beneficial bacteria with the food they need to thrive. It is recommended to consume a variety of prebiotic-rich foods to promote greater bacterial diversity in the intestinal microbiome.

Probiotics for a Balanced Microbiome

Natural Probiotics

Probiotics are living microorganisms, usually beneficial bacteria, that can have positive effects on digestive health and the intestinal microbiome when consumed in adequate amounts. Probiotics contribute to microbiome balance by promoting the growth and activity of beneficial bacteria, inhibiting the proliferation of pathogenic bacteria, and producing beneficial metabolites.

Here are some important facts about natural probiotics:

- Sources of Probiotics: Natural probiotics are mainly found in fermented foods. Common sources of probiotics include yogurt, kefir, sauerkraut, kimchi, miso, tempeh, kombucha, and fermented cheese.

- Beneficial Bacteria: Natural probiotics contain a variety of beneficial bacteria, such as Lactobacillus and Bifidobacterium, which have been associated with positive effects on digestion, immunity, and intestinal health.

- Microbiome Balance: By regularly consuming probiotics, you can help maintain a healthy balance between beneficial bacteria and potentially harmful bacteria in your microbiome.

- Promoting Bacterial Diversity: Probiotics can contribute to bacterial diversity by introducing new strains of bacteria into the microbiome. This can improve the resilience of the microbiome to disturbances.

- Health Benefits: Probiotics have been associated with many health benefits, including regulating digestion, boosting the immune system, reducing inflammation, and supporting mental health.

Artificial Probiotics

Artificial probiotics, also known as probiotic supplements, are beneficial microorganisms cultured in the laboratory and presented in the form of dietary supplements. Unlike natural probiotics found in fermented foods, artificial probiotics are specific strains of bacteria or yeast selected for their probiotic properties.

Here are some important points to know about artificial probiotics:

- Variety of strains: Artificial probiotics are available in several different strains, each with specific health benefits. Some strains are commonly used to support digestive health, while others may have positive effects on immunity, inflammation, or other aspects of health.

- Controlled dosage: Supplemental probiotics allow for precise dosage control, meaning you can choose a specific strain and concentration tailored to your needs.

- Ease of storage: Artificial probiotics are stable and have a longer shelf life than fermented foods, making them convenient to store and use.

- Personalization: Supplemental probiotics may be recommended by a healthcare professional for specific needs. For example, certain probiotic strains may be recommended to treat gastrointestinal disorders such as irritable bowel syndrome or antibiotic-associated diarrhea.

- Precautions: While artificial probiotics are generally considered safe, there may be precautions to consider. Some people may experience mild side effects such as bloating or gastrointestinal issues when taking probiotics. It is important to consult with a healthcare professional before starting a probiotic supplement.

- Synergy with prebiotics: Artificial probiotics can be used in synergy with prebiotics (foods rich in non-digestible fibers) to promote the growth and activity of probiotics in the intestinal microbiome.

- Targeted use: Artificial probiotics are often used in a targeted manner to address specific health issues or to restore balance to the microbiome after disturbances, such as antibiotic use.

It is important to note that artificial probiotics should not replace a diet rich in natural probiotics, but rather complement them. Natural fermented foods offer a wider range of probiotic strains, as well as prebiotics that promote their growth. The combination of fermented foods and supplemental probiotics can contribute to supporting overall microbiome health.

Tips for Incorporating These Foods into Your Daily Diet

Incorporating prebiotics and probiotics into your daily diet may seem daunting, but it can be quite simple by following a few practical tips. Here's how you can integrate these foods into your diet:

- Yogurt for Breakfast: Start your day with a bowl of plain yogurt or kefir. Add fresh fruits, nuts, and honey for a touch of sweetness and flavor.

- Fermented Vegetable Salad: Add fermented vegetables, such as sauerkraut or pickled cucumbers, to your salads for a tangy flavor and probiotic benefits.

- Fruit Smoothies: Make fruit smoothies with yogurt or kefir for a creamy texture and a dose of probiotics.

- Legumes: Incorporate legumes such as lentils, chickpeas, and beans into soups, stews, and stir-fries to benefit from the prebiotics present in these foods.

- Miso in Broths: Use miso paste to add flavor and probiotics to your broths and soups.

- Kefir Cereal: Use kefir instead of milk with your morning cereals for a probiotic boost.

- Yogurt Marinades: Prepare yogurt marinades for meat or chicken. Yogurt helps tenderize the meat while adding delicious flavor.

- Fermented Vegetables as Side Dishes: Serve fermented vegetables, such as kimchi or sauerkraut, as side dishes for main courses, such as sandwiches or burgers.

- Healthy Snacks: Opt for healthy snacks like Greek yogurt with fruits or raw vegetables with hummus for a snack rich in probiotics and prebiotics.

The goal is to make integrating these beneficial foods for your microbiome as simple and delicious as possible. By incorporating them regularly into your daily diet, you contribute to maintaining a balanced microbiome and promote better digestive and immune health.

Conclusion

The fascinating world of microorganisms residing within us plays a crucial role in our health. Dietary diversity, prebiotics, probiotics, and other strategies can help nourish and balance your microbiome, thereby strengthening your immune system. By taking steps to support a healthy microbiome, you can improve your resilience to cancer and your overall well-being.

We will now delve deeper into the role of nutrition during treatments, exploring how specific dietary choices can contribute to supporting resilience and recovery throughout this critical period.

Treatments and Nutrition

Introduction

Let's now enter a domain where nutrition takes on a particularly crucial dimension: the treatment period. In this chapter, we will delve into the importance of a balanced diet during cancer treatments and how it can influence your well-being and your ability to fight the disease.

Cancer treatments, whether it's chemotherapy, radiation therapy, immunotherapy, or other modalities, can exert considerable pressure on the body. It's at this critical moment that nutrition comes into play. Proper nutrition can help meet increased nutritional needs, minimize undesirable side effects, and maintain the strength needed to withstand treatments.

In this chapter, we will thus examine in detail the specific nutritional needs during cancer treatments. You'll discover which foods to prioritize to meet these needs, as well as practical tips for maintaining a balanced diet, even during treatment. We will also address the management of common side effects such as nausea, fatigue, and loss of appetite, to help you navigate through this period as effectively as possible.

Medical consultation and nutritional follow-up will play a key role, and we will guide you on how to collaborate effectively with your medical team to optimize your nutrition during treatments. Additionally, we will explore the role of dietary supplements in this phase, ensuring that they are used appropriately and safely.

This chapter will help you understand why nutrition is an essential element of your cancer treatment plan.

Diet During Treatments

The importance of a balanced diet during cancer treatments is fundamental for several crucial reasons for the well-being and recovery of patients. Here is a detailed explanation of this importance:

- Providing energy and nutrients: Cancer treatments such as chemotherapy, radiation therapy, and surgery can be taxing on the body. They can lead to an increase in energy and nutritional needs. A balanced diet provides the adequate amount of calories, proteins, vitamins, and minerals needed to support healing, repair damaged tissues, and maintain normal bodily function.

- Preventing involuntary weight loss: The disease itself and the side effects of treatments can often result in involuntary weight loss. A balanced diet can help prevent this weight loss by providing essential nutrients and maintaining a healthy body weight. Excessive weight loss can weaken the body and compromise the response to treatment.

- Supporting the immune system: A balanced diet is rich in antioxidants, vitamins, and minerals that play a crucial role in supporting the immune system. A strong immune system is essential for fighting infections and aiding the body in battling cancer. Treatments can weaken the immune system, making it even more important to maintain a healthy diet.

- Managing side effects: Cancer treatments can lead to side effects such as nausea, diarrhea, constipation, fatigue, and loss of appetite. A balanced diet can help alleviate these side effects. For example, eating easily digestible foods can help with gastrointestinal issues, and an energy-rich diet can combat fatigue.

- Promoting healing and recovery: Nutrients from a balanced diet promote healing and recovery after surgeries or aggressive treatments. They help reduce the risk of postoperative complications and speed up recovery.

- Improving treatment tolerance: A balanced diet can help improve treatment tolerance by reducing fatigue, supporting liver function, and minimizing undesirable drug interactions. This can enable patients to better tolerate their treatments.

- Preventing nutritional deficiencies: Cancer treatments can lead to deficiencies in essential nutrients. A balanced diet provides a comprehensive range of nutrients, thus helping to prevent these deficiencies, which are essential for long-term health.

In summary, a balanced diet during cancer treatments helps maintain physical strength, support the immune system, manage side effects, promote healing, and improve treatment tolerance. It is a key element in the journey towards remission and recovery.

Nutritional Needs

The specific nutritional needs during cancer treatments can vary from person to person depending on the type of cancer, stage of the disease, type of treatment (chemotherapy, radiation therapy, immunotherapy, etc.), and the patient's overall health condition. However, some general considerations can be taken into account:

- Proteins: Proteins are essential for tissue repair, maintaining muscle mass, and immune function. Cancer patients may have an increased need for proteins due to the disease and treatments. Lean protein sources such as lean meats, fish, eggs, low-fat dairy products, legumes, and nuts can help meet these needs.

- Calories: Cancer treatments and the disease itself can increase the body's calorie needs. It is important to maintain adequate calorie intake to prevent involuntary weight loss, but this should be done in a balanced manner to avoid excessive weight gain.

- Hydration: Dehydration can be a common side effect of cancer treatments, especially chemotherapy. It is essential to stay well-hydrated to support kidney function and minimize adverse effects. Drinking enough water, unsweetened beverages, and herbal teas is important.

- Fiber: Dietary fiber can help prevent constipation, a common side effect of cancer treatments and certain medications. Vegetables, fruits, legumes, and whole grains are good sources of fiber.

- Vitamins and minerals: Some vitamins and minerals may become depleted during treatments, including vitamin D, calcium, iron, and B vitamins. It may be necessary to take supplements under the supervision of a healthcare professional to address these nutritional gaps.

- Antioxidants: Antioxidants found in fruits and vegetables can help combat free radicals produced during cancer treatments. They are important for immune support and cellular health.

- Infection prevention: A balanced diet rich in proteins and essential nutrients can help strengthen the immune system and prevent infections, which are often more common in cancer patients.

It is important to note that nutritional needs may change throughout the course of treatment and recovery. Therefore, patients are recommended to work closely with a nutritionist to develop a personalized plan based on their health status and specific needs. Regular monitoring throughout treatment can help adjust the nutritional plan accordingly. The goal is to support the body in its fight against cancer while improving the quality of life during this challenging period.

Foods to Prioritize

During cancer treatments, it is essential to prioritize foods that support health, boost the immune system, and help reduce side effects. Here is a list of foods to prioritize in your diet during this period:

- Leafy green vegetables: Leafy greens such as spinach, kale, romaine lettuce, and broccoli are rich in vitamins, minerals, fiber, and antioxidants. They help strengthen the immune system and fight cellular damage.

- Fresh fruits: Fruits such as berries, citrus fruits, apples, and pears provide a variety of vitamins, minerals, and antioxidants. Fruits are also a natural source of sugar for an energy boost.

- Lean proteins: Lean protein sources such as skinless chicken, turkey, fish, eggs, and legumes are essential for tissue repair, maintaining muscle mass, and recovery.

- Whole grains: Whole grains like brown rice, oats, quinoa, and whole wheat are rich in fiber and provide sustained energy, which can help combat fatigue.

- Legumes: Beans, lentils, chickpeas, and peas are excellent sources of plant-based proteins, fiber, and essential nutrients. They help maintain a balanced diet.

- Low-fat dairy products: Low-fat dairy products such as yogurt and milk provide calcium and proteins. If you are lactose intolerant, opt for lactose-free alternatives like almond or soy milk.

- Omega-3-rich foods: Fatty fish such as salmon, mackerel, sardines, and nuts are rich in omega-3 fatty acids, which have anti-inflammatory properties and can help reduce inflammation.

- Iron-rich foods: If you have anemia, include iron-rich foods in your diet, such as spinach, lentils, lean meat, and fortified cereals.

- Antioxidant-rich foods: Antioxidant-rich foods like berries, tomatoes, carrots, green tea, and nuts help neutralize free radicals and protect cells from damage.

By prioritizing these foods in your diet, you provide your body with essential nutrients needed to maintain your energy, strength, and resilience during cancer treatments. Also, make sure to stay well-hydrated by drinking enough water throughout the day to support your optimal functioning.

Practical Tips

Here are some practical tips for meal planning during this period:

- Eat regularly: Try to eat every few hours to maintain adequate calorie intake and avoid fatigue. If you experience nausea or appetite problems, consider eating smaller portions throughout the day rather than three large meals. Nutritious snacks can also be helpful.

- Choose easily digestible foods: Opt for foods that are gentle on the stomach and digestive system. Cooked foods, such as steamed vegetables, cooked grains, soups, and purees, may be easier to tolerate than raw or spicy foods.

- Stay well-hydrated: Drink plenty of water to prevent dehydration, especially if you experience diarrhea or vomiting. Unsweetened herbal teas and electrolyte drinks can help maintain hydration.

- Avoid trigger foods: If certain foods trigger nausea, acid reflux, or other gastrointestinal issues, try to temporarily avoid them.

Managing Side Effects

Strategies for Nausea

Nausea is one of the most common side effects of cancer treatments. Here are some strategies to manage it:

- Easy-to-digest foods: Opt for light, easy-to-digest foods such as salted crackers, oatmeal, white rice, baked apples, or applesauce.

- Meal fractioning: Eat smaller portions more frequently throughout the day to avoid overloading your stomach.

- Avoid strong smells: Stay away from foods or scents that trigger nausea. Good ventilation in the kitchen can also help.

- Ginger: Ginger, in the form of tea, ginger candies, or ginger capsules, may help relieve nausea for some people.

- Medications: If nausea is severe, your doctor may prescribe anti-nausea medications. Make sure to take them as directed.

Appetite Stimulation

Loss of appetite is a common challenge during cancer treatments. Here are some tips to stimulate appetite:

- Eat small amounts frequently: Instead of three large meals, try eating several small nutritious snacks throughout the day.

- Choose calorie-rich foods: Opt for calorie and nutrient-rich foods such as fruit smoothies, nuts, cheese, avocados, and eggs.

- Vary flavors: Experiment with different flavors and textures to avoid food monotony. Try sweet, savory, sour, and spicy dishes.

- Drink liquids between meals: Avoid drinking too many liquids during meals to prevent feeling too full. Instead, drink between meals to maintain hydration.

- Focus on enjoyed foods: Focus on foods that you really enjoy. This can help make meals more appealing.

Weight Loss

Involuntary weight loss can be concerning during treatments. Here are some strategies to manage it:

- Calorie-rich foods: Choose calorie and nutrient-rich foods such as nuts, avocados, full-fat dairy products, and whole grains.

- Nutritional supplements: Your doctor or nutritionist may recommend nutritional supplements to increase your calorie intake.

- Proteins: Make sure to consume enough proteins to prevent muscle loss. Lean protein sources such as chicken, fish, and eggs are important.

Managing Fatigue

Fatigue is a common side effect of cancer treatments. A balanced diet can help manage fatigue by providing a steady source of energy. Make sure to:

- Eat regularly: Avoid prolonged fasting by eating regularly throughout the day.

- Choose complex carbohydrates: Whole grains, legumes, and vegetables provide sustained energy and can help combat fatigue.

- Avoid refined sugar: Blood sugar spikes and crashes can worsen fatigue. Avoid foods high in refined sugar.

Gastrointestinal Side Effects

To minimize gastrointestinal problems such as diarrhea or constipation, it is essential to choose foods suitable for your digestive tolerance. Avoid spicy, fatty, or irritating foods for your stomach, and opt for easy-to-digest foods such as cooked cereals, cooked vegetables, and foods rich in soluble fiber.

Consultation and Nutritional Follow-Up

Medical consultation and nutritional follow-up play a crucial role in managing nutrition during cancer treatments. Here's why it's essential to consult a healthcare professional or a nutritionist specialized in cancer:

- Individual assessment: Everyone responds differently to treatments and side effects. An individual assessment of your health status, nutritional needs, and food preferences is necessary to develop a dietary plan tailored to your situation.

- Side effect management: A healthcare professional can help you manage these side effects by adjusting your diet and recommending nutritional supplements if necessary.

- Prevention of deficiencies: Cancer treatments can increase your body's nutritional needs. It's essential to ensure that you're getting enough nutrients to maintain your health and vitality. A nutritionist can monitor your nutrient intake and recommend supplements if deficiencies are identified.

- Emotional support: Cancer and its treatments can have a significant emotional impact. A healthcare professional can provide emotional support by helping you cope with food-related challenges and maintain a positive attitude towards nutrition.

- Follow-up and adjustments: Your nutritional plan needs to be flexible to adapt to changes during treatments. Regular follow-up with a healthcare professional will allow for adjustments as needed to optimize your well-being.

- Prevention and recovery: A balanced diet during treatments can contribute to preventing complications and faster recovery. Proper nutritional follow-up can also play a role in preventing cancer recurrence.

In summary, consulting a healthcare professional or a nutritionist specialized in cancer is essential to ensure that your diet meets your specific needs during treatments. This can help improve your quality of life, minimize undesirable side effects, and support your body in its fight against the disease. Don't hesitate to ask questions, express your concerns, and collaborate closely with your medical team to ensure comprehensive management of your health.

Dietary Supplements

Importance of Supplements

Dietary supplements can play a crucial role in overall health management during cancer treatments. Here's why their use can be beneficial:

- Nutritional support: Cancer treatments can increase the body's nutritional needs due to side effects such as loss of appetite, nausea, and weight loss. Dietary supplements can help fill nutritional gaps and provide essential nutrients needed to maintain health.

- Reduction of side effects: Some supplements, such as antioxidants, can help reduce treatment side effects such as fatigue, nausea, and cellular damage. They act by neutralizing free radicals, which are produced in excess during treatments.

- Immune system strengthening: Some supplements, like vitamin D, zinc, and selenium, are known to strengthen the immune system. A strong immune system can help fight infections and support the body's response to treatments.

- Improvement of quality of life: Supplements can contribute to improving the quality of life by reducing symptoms such as fatigue, excessive weight loss, and weakness, allowing patients to better tolerate treatments.

Recommended Supplements

Essential vitamins:

- Vitamin D plays a crucial role in bone and immune health. It is particularly important during treatments as it can help prevent bone loss and strengthen the immune system.

- Vitamin C is a powerful antioxidant that can help reduce side effects such as fatigue and support the immune system.

Minerals and trace elements:

- Zinc is necessary for wound healing, immune function, and appetite regulation. It can be helpful for patients experiencing loss of appetite.

- Selenium is a mineral with antioxidant properties and can help protect cells from damage caused by treatments.

Antioxidants:

- Flavonoids and carotenoids are antioxidants found in many fruits and vegetables. They can help reduce inflammation and minimize treatment side effects.

Interaction with Treatments

It is important to note that some supplements may interact with cancer treatments. For example, some antioxidants may neutralize the effects of chemotherapy agents, reducing their effectiveness. That's why it's essential to consult a healthcare professional before taking supplements during treatments. Your medical team can advise you on appropriate supplements, their dosage, and the optimal timing to avoid undesirable interactions.

Conclusion

In this chapter, we've seen how proper nutrition can help manage treatment side effects, maintain strength and vitality, and support the healing process. Thus, nutrition should be an integral part of your overall treatment plan. By taking steps to meet your nutritional needs during this time, you can improve your tolerance to treatments and your quality of life.

We will now explore the role of calorie restriction and fasting for tailored nutrition during treatments, active prevention, and sustainable healing.

Calorie Restriction and Fasting

Introduction

As our exploration of anticancer nutrition continues, we delve into an exciting and controversial area of research: calorie restriction and fasting. In this chapter, we will examine these dietary practices in-depth and their potential in cancer prevention and treatment.

Calorie restriction, which involves deliberately reducing calorie intake, and fasting, which involves periods of food deprivation, have garnered increasing interest in the field of health. Many studies have suggested that these approaches could have potential benefits, particularly concerning treatment sensitivity and protection of healthy cells during cancer treatments.

In this chapter, we will delve into the underlying principles of calorie restriction and fasting. You will discover the potential benefits of these practices, including their impact on treatment tolerance, their ability to protect healthy cells, and their potential to sensitize cancer cells.

We will also examine the different types of fasting and common practices, as well as the potential risks associated with these approaches. Our goal is to provide you with comprehensive and balanced information so that you can make informed decisions in the context of cancer treatment.

Basic Principles

Fasting and calorie restriction are two related approaches that involve reducing food consumption, but they have distinct characteristics. Understanding these principles is essential for considering their potential use in cancer prevention and treatment.

Fasting

Fasting is a dietary practice that involves abstaining from eating for a determined period. It can be practiced in various ways, including intermittent fasting, water fasting, and dry fasting. Intermittent fasting involves alternating periods of fasting and meals, while water fasting involves abstaining from all solid food, consuming only water. Dry fasting, on the other hand, allows neither food nor liquids.

Fasting can be used for various reasons, including weight loss, improving insulin sensitivity, cell regeneration, reducing inflammation, and promoting autophagy, a cellular cleansing process. Some studies suggest that fasting may also have potential effects in cancer prevention by reducing risk factors such as inflammation and high insulin levels.

Calorie Restriction

Calorie restriction involves a deliberate reduction in daily calorie intake, typically without imposing strict fasting periods. Instead, it entails reducing the total amount of calories consumed while ensuring a balanced diet in terms of essential nutrients.

Calorie restriction has been studied for its potential effects on longevity and reducing the risk of age-related diseases, including cancer. Some research has shown that calorie restriction can positively influence metabolic and hormonal processes that contribute to overall health. However, it's important to note that calorie restriction should be practiced thoughtfully, under medical supervision if necessary, to avoid nutritional deficiencies and adverse effects.

Thus, the potential use of fasting and calorie restriction in cancer prevention and treatment is based on the idea that these approaches can influence risk factors such as inflammation, high insulin, and cellular regeneration. However, it's essential to understand that these practices are not suitable for everyone, and they should be approached with caution, in consultation with a healthcare professional.

Potential Benefits

Cellular Regeneration

Fasting and calorie restriction can promote cellular regeneration, a crucial process for health. When we fast or reduce our calorie intake, our body undergoes a process called autophagy. Autophagy is a cellular cleansing mechanism in which cells break down and remove damaged or obsolete cellular components.

This cleansing process helps eliminate cellular debris, faulty proteins, and damaged mitochondrial components. It also promotes the regeneration of new healthy cells. By promoting autophagy, fasting can contribute to DNA repair, reducing cancer-related risk factors, and slowing cellular aging.

Reduction of Inflammation

Chronic inflammation is a risk factor for many diseases, including cancer. Fasting and calorie restriction can help reduce inflammation in the body.

When we fast, our body reduces the production of pro-inflammatory molecules. Additionally, intermittent fasting may promote the production of adiponectin, a hormone with anti-inflammatory properties. Fasting can also reduce levels of interleukin-6 (IL-6), a pro-inflammatory cytokine. By reducing inflammation, fasting and calorie restriction can help prevent some inflammation-related diseases, including cancer.

Improvement of Insulin Sensitivity

Insulin is a crucial hormone that regulates blood sugar levels and how cells use glucose as an energy source. Reduced insulin sensitivity is associated with high insulin levels in the blood, which can promote the growth of cancer cells.

Fasting and calorie restriction can improve insulin sensitivity. During fasting periods, the body utilizes glucose stored in the liver and muscles, which can reduce insulin resistance. Additionally, these approaches can stimulate the production of adiponectin, which promotes glucose utilization by cells.

Types of Fasting and Common Practices

Different types of fasting and calorie restriction have specific characteristics. Here's a detailed explanation of these common practices:

Intermittent Fasting

Intermittent fasting has become one of the most popular approaches in anticancer nutrition. It involves alternating between periods of fasting and periods of eating. The most common methods of intermittent fasting are as follows:

- 16/8 fasting: This is one of the most popular methods, where you fast for 16 hours a day and have an 8-hour eating window. For example, you might eat between 12 pm and 8 pm and fast for the rest of the time.

- 5:2 fasting: It involves eating normally for five days of the week and significantly reducing calories (about 500-600 calories) for two fasting days.

- Alternate-day fasting: You alternate between full fasting days and normal eating days.

Water Fasting

Water fasting is a more intense practice that involves abstaining from eating any solid food and consuming only water for a set period. Water fasts can vary in duration, ranging from a few hours to several days. They should be done with caution and under medical supervision for prolonged fasts.

Dry Fasting

Dry fasting is the most extreme form of fasting, where no food or liquids, including water, are consumed. It is generally not recommended due to the risks associated with dehydration and potential complications.

Calorie Restriction

Calorie restriction involves deliberately reducing daily calorie intake while maintaining a balanced diet. This can be achieved by consuming fewer calories than the body normally burns in a day.

Role of Fasting during Treatments

Fasting during cancer treatments is gaining interest due to its potential health benefits. Here's a more detailed exploration of its role during treatments:

Treatment Tolerance

Fasting may help reduce treatment-induced nausea and vomiting by reducing irritation of the gastrointestinal mucosa and regulating the release of certain chemicals involved in these symptoms.

Fasting may also help combat fatigue by stimulating the production of certain molecules that enhance cellular energy and by reducing systemic inflammation that can contribute to fatigue.

Cell Protection

Fasting can act as a protective factor for healthy cells during treatments by preparing them to better withstand damage from aggressive treatments. At the same time, it may sensitize cancer cells by disrupting their anaerobic (glucose-dependent) metabolism and making them more receptive to treatments. This sensitization could potentially improve the effectiveness of anticancer therapies.

Some preliminary studies conducted on animal models have shown that intermittent fasting may also slow tumor progression, reduce their size, and in some cases, improve response to anticancer treatments. However, these results need to be confirmed by clinical studies on humans.

Potential Risks

While fasting may present potential benefits in cancer treatment, it is crucial to understand and consider the associated risks. Here are some potential risks of fasting to be taken into account:

- Excessive Weight Loss: Prolonged fasting, especially if not properly supervised, can lead to excessive weight loss, which can be concerning for individuals already weakened by cancer or its treatments.

- Dehydration: Fasting can increase the risk of dehydration, especially if fluid intake is inadequate. Dehydration can worsen the side effects of cancer treatments.

- Electrolyte Imbalances: Prolonged fasting can result in electrolyte imbalances, such as abnormally low levels of sodium, potassium, or other essential electrolytes, which can have serious health consequences.

- Fatigue and Weakness: Fasting can lead to increased fatigue and feelings of weakness, which can be particularly challenging for individuals already fatigued by cancer treatments.

- Medical Side Effects: Fasting can interact with certain medications or treatments, leading to undesirable medical side effects. It is essential to consult a healthcare professional to assess these potential interactions.

- Risk of Malnutrition: Unsupervised fasting can lead to malnutrition as it limits the intake of essential nutrients. This can further weaken the immune system and compromise the body's ability to fight cancer.

- Psychological Effects: Fasting can have psychological effects, such as anxiety, frustration, and depression, especially if individuals feel compelled to fast or meet certain expectations.

It is imperative to remember that fasting is not suitable for everyone. Before starting a fasting program, it is strongly recommended to consult a healthcare professional, preferably an oncologist or a oncology specialized nutritionist. They can assess the individual situation, nutritional needs, and potential risks, and recommend the best approach for each person. Fasting should always be conducted under medical supervision to minimize risks and optimize potential benefits.

Conclusion

In this chapter, we have explored the principles and practices related to fasting and calorie restriction and their potential impact on cancer prevention and treatment. We have examined the potential benefits, types of fasting, as well as precautions and associated risks. They can be powerful tools to improve treatment response and strengthen the body's ability to fight cancer. However, it is essential to approach them with caution and under appropriate supervision.

We will now address the theme of recurrence. Understanding this complex phenomenon is of great importance as it can have a significant impact on patients' lives and treatment decisions.

Preventing Recurrence

Introduction

In this chapter, we will delve deep into nutritional strategies and lifestyle choices that can play a key role in building a strong defense against cancer recurrence.

Cancer recurrence is a major concern for many individuals who have already faced this disease. However, it is crucial to understand that nutrition and lifestyle can actively contribute to preventing this possibility. By building a strong defense against recurrence, you can enhance your long-term health and well-being.

In this chapter, we will explore in detail specific nutritional strategies for preventing recurrence. You will discover the importance of maintaining a healthy and balanced diet to support your body in its fight against potentially residual cancer cells.

We will also address the importance of balance and overall well-being in long-term prevention. Health is not limited to what's on your plate, and we'll explore how stress, physical activity, and other lifestyle factors can influence your ability to prevent recurrence.

Prevention Strategies

Preventing Recurrence

The importance of prevention in the fight against cancer recurrence is invaluable. It constitutes an essential pillar for reducing the risks of relapse and improving the quality of life of patients by promoting healthy lifestyles, regular medical follow-up, and risk factor management. By focusing on prevention, we can not only reduce the likelihood of recurrence but also contribute to the long-term health of cancer survivors.

Thus, prevention in this context primarily aims to reduce the risks of developing a new tumor after an initial episode of cancer or seeing cancer return after initial treatment. Here's why prevention is crucial in this fight:

- Reducing the Risk of Recurrence: Prevention primarily aims to reduce the risk factors that can promote cancer recurrence. By adopting a healthy lifestyle, monitoring one's diet, avoiding risky behaviors (such as smoking), and following medical recommendations, one can minimize the chances of cancer returning.

- Improving Quality of Life: Cancer treatments, such as surgery, chemotherapy, and radiotherapy, can have debilitating side effects. Prevention aims to avoid undergoing these treatments again, which can greatly improve the quality of life of cancer survivors.

- Saving Healthcare Resources: Cancer recurrence often requires costly and resource-intensive treatments. By preventing recurrence, we contribute to saving these resources, which can be beneficial for both the healthcare system and patients.

- Patient Empowerment: Prevention empowers cancer survivors to take control of their own health. By understanding risk factors and adopting a healthy lifestyle, patients feel more involved in their healing journey and have better control over their health.

Healthy Diet to Prevent Recurrence

Preventing cancer recurrence is a major concern for individuals who have survived an initial episode of the disease. Diet plays a crucial role in this prevention as it can help maintain an environment in the body that is less conducive to the growth of cancer cells. Here are some nutritional strategies to prevent cancer recurrence:

- Maintain a Healthy Body Weight: Maintaining a healthy body weight is crucial for preventing cancer recurrence. Obesity is a major risk factor for cancer, and weight loss can help reduce this risk. A balanced diet rich in vegetables, fruits, whole grains, and lean proteins, combined with regular physical activity, can help maintain a healthy body weight.

- Adopt an Anti-inflammatory Diet: Chronic inflammation is linked to cancer development. An anti-inflammatory diet, rich in foods such as colorful fruits and vegetables, legumes, nuts, seeds, and fatty fish, can help reduce inflammation in the body.

- Limit Consumption of Processed Foods: Processed foods, high in added sugars, trans fats, and additives, can promote inflammation and increase the risk of cancer recurrence. It is essential to limit their consumption.

- Embrace Superfoods: Superfoods, rich in antioxidants, phytonutrients, and vitamins, can boost the immune system and help prevent cancer recurrence. Cruciferous vegetables (broccoli, cauliflower), berries, spinach, turmeric, and garlic are some examples of superfoods.

- Opt for Healthy Fats: Healthy fats, such as those found in olive oil, avocados, nuts, and fatty fish, can help reduce inflammation and maintain an environment in the body that is unfavorable for cancer.

- Limit Alcohol Consumption: Excessive alcohol consumption is associated with an increased risk of cancer recurrence. It is recommended to limit alcohol consumption or avoid it altogether.

- Monitor Sugar Intake: Limiting the consumption of added sugars, especially in sugary beverages and sweetened products, can help maintain stable blood sugar levels, which is important for preventing cancer recurrence.

- Restrict Consumption of Red and Processed Meats: Red and processed meats, such as bacon and sausages, are associated with an increased risk of cancer. It is recommended to consume them in moderation.

Thus, a balanced diet rich in anti-inflammatory foods, superfoods, and healthy fats, combined with proper weight management and regular medical follow-up, can significantly contribute to preventing cancer recurrence. It is essential to work closely with healthcare professionals to develop a nutrition plan tailored to each individual.

Balance and Moderation

Moderation is Essential

Avoiding Over-Restriction in Diet

It is essential to understand that preventing cancer recurrence does not require over-restriction in diet. Indeed, adopting an extremely strict and restrictive diet can not only be challenging to sustain in the long term but also harmful to mental and physical health.

While it is true that preventing cancer recurrence partly relies on healthy dietary choices, it does not mean that one must deprive oneself of all culinary pleasures. Over-restriction in diet can be stressful and lead to anxiety, which, in turn, can have negative effects on the immune system and overall well-being. Therefore, it is important to find a balance between maintaining a healthy diet and occasionally indulging in favorite foods, even if they are not necessarily the most nutritious.

Moderation and Variety

Moderation and variety are key principles for a balanced diet and an effective strategy for preventing cancer recurrence. Moderation involves consuming nutrient-rich foods while avoiding excess, while variety means including a wide range of foods in one's diet.

By adopting a balanced approach, you can reap the benefits of different types of foods, each providing its own essential nutrients. For example, vegetables provide a variety of vitamins and minerals, lean proteins are essential for cell repair, healthy fats support heart health, and complex carbohydrates provide sustained energy.

By including a variety of foods in your diet, you are more likely to meet your nutritional needs and maintain a diet that is both nourishing and enjoyable. This approach also promotes a healthier relationship with food, eliminating the guilt associated with occasional consumption of less healthy foods.

Ultimately, it is important to remember that preventing cancer recurrence does not require total deprivation but rather a balanced approach. This allows for maintaining a healthy diet while preserving the pleasure of eating, which is essential for a balanced and fulfilling life.

Diet, Exercise, and Mental Well-being

Importance of Balance

Balancing diet, exercise, and mental well-being is a fundamental pillar for optimal health and the prevention of cancer recurrence. These three aspects of our lives are closely interconnected and mutually reinforcing.

Diet provides essential nutrients that our body needs to function properly, support the immune system, and prevent inflammation. It also plays a key role in weight management, an important factor in cancer recurrence prevention.

Regular exercise not only helps maintain a healthy body weight but also has positive effects on mental health. Physical activity releases endorphins, chemicals that promote a sense of well-being and reduce stress, anxiety, and depression. Moreover, exercise strengthens the immune system and promotes better blood circulation, which is essential for nutrient transport.

Mental well-being is as important as diet and exercise for preventing cancer recurrence. Chronic stress, anxiety, and depression can negatively impact the immune system and promote inflammation, potentially contributing to cancer progression. Stress management, mindfulness practice, and relaxation techniques are effective ways to support mental health.

Stress Management

Stress management is a key element of mental well-being. Here are some practical tips for effectively managing stress:

- Practice meditation and mindfulness: Regular meditation can help calm the mind, reduce anxiety, and improve concentration. Mindfulness allows you to stay present in the moment.

- Exercise regularly: Physical exercise is an excellent way to reduce stress. Choose an activity you enjoy, whether it's walking, running, yoga, or dancing, and practice it regularly.

- Prioritize sleep: Quality sleep is essential for stress management. Establish a regular sleep routine and create a conducive environment for rest.

- Talk about your feelings: Don't keep your emotions to yourself. Talk to a friend, family member, or mental health professional about how you're feeling.

- Avoid unnecessary stressors: Identify sources of stress in your life and try to minimize them as much as possible. This may include time management, task delegation, or changing your environment.

Hydration and Sleep

Importance of Hydration

Hydration is an essential aspect of health and cancer recurrence prevention. Water plays many vital roles in the human body, and maintaining it at an optimal level is crucial for optimal functioning. Here's why hydration is so important:

- Role in digestion and nutrient absorption: Water is necessary for digesting food and absorbing essential nutrients. It facilitates the transport of nutrients through the digestive tract to the cells that need them.

- Toxin elimination: Water helps eliminate waste and toxins from the body through urine, sweat, and stools. Adequate hydration ensures an efficient elimination system.

- Maintenance of electrolyte balance: Water is essential for maintaining the balance of electrolytes in the body, including sodium, potassium, and magnesium. This balance is crucial for cellular health and regulating blood pressure.

- Body temperature regulation: Water helps regulate body temperature by absorbing heat generated during physical activity and releasing it through sweating.

To maintain adequate hydration, it is recommended to drink about 8 glasses of water per day, although individual needs may vary depending on age, activity level, and weather conditions. Hydration is not limited to pure water only; fruit juices, unsweetened herbal teas, and water-rich foods like fruits and vegetables also contribute to fluid intake.

The Crucial Role of Sleep

Quality sleep is another key element in cancer recurrence prevention. During sleep, the body performs many functions of regeneration and cellular repair. Here's why sleep is crucial for overall health:

- Cellular repair: During sleep, cells have the opportunity to repair and regenerate. This includes repairing damaged DNA, which can be a factor in cancer prevention.

- Immune system strengthening: Quality sleep is essential for the proper functioning of the immune system. A strong immune system can better detect and fight cancer cells.

- Stress reduction: Sleep contributes to reducing stress, anxiety, and depression, which are essential for mental and emotional health.

- Hormonal balance: Sleep regulates the production of hormones, including those related to hunger and satiety. Inadequate sleep can disrupt these hormones and contribute to weight gain.

To improve the quality of your sleep, it is recommended to maintain a regular sleep routine, avoid caffeine and electronic screens before bedtime, and create a comfortable and dark sleep environment. The amount of sleep needed varies by age, but generally, adults need 7 to 9 hours of sleep per night for optimal health.

Regular Physical Activity and Risk Reduction

The Benefits of Physical Activity

Regular physical activity offers numerous health benefits and can help reduce the risk of recurrence. Here are some of the benefits of physical activity in the context of cancer recurrence prevention:

- Strengthening the immune system: Regular exercise can boost the immune system by increasing the production of immune cells, enabling the body to better fight potential cancer cells.

- Reducing inflammation: Chronic inflammation is a risk factor for cancer and recurrence. Exercise can help reduce inflammation in the body.

- Weight management: Physical activity helps maintain a healthy body weight. Obesity is associated with an increased risk of cancer recurrence in many cases.

- Improving heart and lung function: Regular exercise improves heart and lung function, which can be particularly important during and after cancer treatments.

- Reducing stress and anxiety: Physical activity releases endorphins, feel-good hormones, which can help reduce stress and anxiety, thereby improving mental health.

- Enhancing quality of life: Exercise can contribute to an overall better quality of life by boosting fitness, increasing energy, and improving mobility.

Tips for Reducing Risk Factors

Reducing cancer-related risk factors is another essential component of recurrence prevention. Here are some tips for reducing these risk factors:

- Smoking: If you smoke, seriously consider quitting. Smoking is a major risk factor for cancer, and quitting smoking can significantly reduce this risk.

- Alcohol consumption: Limit alcohol consumption, as alcohol abuse is associated with an increased risk of certain types of cancer.

- Sun protection: Use adequate sun protection to reduce the risk of skin cancer.

- Medical screening: Regularly undergo appropriate cancer screening tests based on your age and gender. Early detection can improve chances of recovery.

Conclusion

In this chapter dedicated to cancer recurrence prevention, we have explored essential strategies for maintaining a long-term anticancer lifestyle. We have discussed the importance of healthy dietary choices and emphasized the crucial role of balance and well-being in this quest. By adopting a sustainable anticancer lifestyle, you can contribute to reducing the risks of recurrence and improving your quality of life.

Now, we will delve into the latest scientific advancements that can illuminate our path. We will explore the latest findings to better understand ways to optimize the prevention and management of this complex disease.

Advancements and Perspectives

Introduction

In this chapter, we will explore the latest recent advancements and perspectives for the future. Medical science continues to progress, opening new avenues in cancer prevention, diagnosis, and treatment. Researchers worldwide are tirelessly working to understand this complex disease and develop more effective approaches. Here, we will address the essential role of nutrition and complementary therapies in this constantly evolving medical research context.

Reflection on Progress Made

Assessment of Anticancer Nutrition Advancements

Over the decades, research in anticancer nutrition has seen significant advancements that have led to a better understanding of how diet can play a crucial role in cancer prevention and treatment. Here are some of the major advancements in anticancer nutrition:

- Identification of Superfoods: Research has identified superfoods rich in antioxidants, phytonutrients, vitamins, and minerals, which have shown their ability to protect cells against damage and strengthen the immune system.

- Understanding Mechanisms: Scientists have discovered how certain food compounds, such as green tea polyphenols or soy isoflavones, can influence cellular mechanisms related to tumor growth and inflammation.

- Epidemiological Studies: Large-scale studies have established links between certain dietary patterns and the risk of cancer, including the Mediterranean diet, which has been shown to be protective.

- Advancements in Supplements: Specific dietary supplements, such as probiotics, prebiotics, and certain nutrients, have been studied for their potential role in supporting health during cancer and treatments.

Impact on Prevention and Treatment

These advancements in anticancer nutrition have had a significant impact on cancer prevention and treatment. Here's how they have influenced these areas:

- Prevention: Anticancer nutrition recommendations have become more precise, helping individuals make informed decisions about their diet. Diets rich in superfoods, antioxidants, and essential nutrients are now recommended to reduce the risk of cancer.

- Treatment: As part of cancer treatment, an appropriate diet can help minimize the side effects of treatments, support the immune system, and improve the quality of life for patients. Specific dietary supplements are sometimes used to alleviate symptoms.

Promising Research Areas

Personalized Medicine

Personalized medicine is a research area that holds immense potential in the field of anticancer nutrition. It is based on the idea that each individual is unique, and therefore, their response to diet may vary depending on their genetic characteristics, metabolism, and specific risk factors.

In the context of anticancer nutrition, personalized medicine allows for a better understanding of how certain foods and nutrients interact with individual genes, potentially influencing the risk of cancer, treatment response, and prevention of recurrence. Studies are underway to identify genetic and metabolic biomarkers that could help personalize dietary recommendations.

For example, if a person has a genetic predisposition to a specific type of cancer, they could benefit from tailored nutrition to reduce their risk. Similarly, personalized medicine can help choose the most appropriate dietary supplements based on an individual's genetic profile.

Immunotherapy

Immunotherapy is a major breakthrough in cancer treatment. It involves stimulating the patient's immune system to recognize and destroy cancer cells. Immunotherapy has revolutionized the management of certain cancers and offers new perspectives in the fight against the disease.

Nutrition plays a crucial role in supporting the immune system, and this is where the link between immunotherapy and anticancer nutrition lies. Research is underway to understand how diet can be optimized to enhance the effectiveness of immunotherapy.

Some substances found in foods, such as beta-glucans in mushrooms, polyphenols in berries, or probiotics, may impact immunity and response to immunotherapy treatments. Studies are seeking to determine how to integrate these foods and dietary supplements into the diet of patients undergoing immunotherapy to improve their treatment response.

Complementary Therapies

Combining Nutrition and Complementary Therapies

The combination of nutrition with other complementary therapies is a rapidly expanding field of research and practice in the fight against cancer. This holistic approach aims to integrate specific nutritional interventions with other treatment methods, such as traditional medicine, complementary and alternative therapies, psycho-oncology, functional medicine, etc.

The goal of this combination is to maximize benefits for the patient by adopting a multidimensional approach. For example, a cancer patient may benefit from chemotherapy or radiotherapy in combination with a targeted diet rich in antioxidants and specific nutrients that can help reduce side effects and support treatment response.

Additionally, approaches such as acupuncture, meditation, massage therapy, and other complementary therapies can be integrated to help manage stress, pain, nausea, and other symptoms associated with cancer treatment.

Combining nutrition with complementary therapies can also contribute to improving patients' quality of life and strengthening their immune system. However, it is essential that this approach be supervised by a team of healthcare professionals, including oncologists, nutritionists, and other specialists, to ensure the safety and effectiveness of the entire treatment plan.

Advancements in Dietary Supplements

Dietary supplements are an important component of anticancer nutrition. Advances in this field focus on the search for new substances, formulations, and combinations of nutrients that can help prevent cancer recurrence and improve patients' quality of life.

Some recent advancements include the development of dietary supplements specifically designed for the nutritional needs of cancer patients, taking into account their treatments and symptoms. For example, supplements enriched with antioxidants, omega-3 fatty acids, vitamins, and minerals may be recommended to help combat fatigue, nausea, and common nutritional deficiencies in patients undergoing treatment.

Furthermore, research is ongoing to identify new natural compounds found in plants, seaweed, mushrooms, etc., that may have potential anticancer properties. These compounds are then used to develop specific dietary supplements aimed at boosting the immune system, reducing inflammation, and supporting the healing process.

Advancements in dietary supplements also aim to better understand nutrient interactions, determine optimal dosages, and ensure the quality and safety of products available on the market.

Ultimately, these advancements in dietary supplements contribute to expanding options available for cancer patients and optimizing the nutritional approach in the prevention of recurrence and treatment of the disease.

Challenges to Overcome

Complexity of Research

Research in anticancer nutrition is a complex field that presents many challenges to researchers and healthcare professionals. Here are some of the main challenges associated with this field:

- Individual Variability: Each individual reacts differently to foods and nutrients, depending on factors such as genetic heritage, age, gender, metabolism, medical history, and more. This variability makes it difficult to create universal nutritional recommendations for cancer prevention and treatment.

- Complexity of Interactions: Foods and nutrients interact in complex ways within the body, making it difficult to understand the exact mechanisms by which they can influence cancer growth. For example, some nutrients may have protective effects when consumed together but not when taken separately.

- Need for Solid Evidence: Establishing a causal link between nutrition and cancer requires strong scientific evidence, usually obtained from large-scale longitudinal studies and controlled clinical trials. Data collection over a long period and the follow-up of patient cohorts are costly and time-consuming processes.

- Influence of Environmental Factors: Dietary habits and exposure to environmental carcinogens such as air pollution, food toxins, smoking, and radiation exposure can play a major role in cancer development. Distinguishing the effects of nutrition from other risk factors can be challenging.

- Different Types of Cancer: There are many types of cancer, each with its own characteristics and mechanisms. What may be beneficial for the prevention or treatment of one type of cancer may not be so for another, making research even more complex.

Education and Awareness

Education and public awareness of effective anticancer nutrition are essential for promoting healthy dietary choices and reducing the risk of cancer. Here are some of the challenges to overcome in this context:

- Misinformation: There is a lot of contradictory and often unfounded information about nutrition and cancer. Myths and misconceptions can blur the public's understanding of healthy dietary choices.

- Complexity of Nutrition: Nutrition is a complex and constantly evolving field. Nutritional recommendations can be difficult for the general public to understand. Effective education should simplify concepts while providing accurate information.

- Cultural and Social Challenges: Dietary habits are strongly influenced by culture, food availability, the economy, and other social factors. Raising awareness about anticancer nutrition while respecting these factors is a challenge.

Targeted educational campaigns, online resources, workshops, and school-based education programs can help increase awareness of effective anticancer nutrition.

Healthcare professionals also play a crucial role in nutrition education. They can provide personalized, evidence-based information to their patients, helping them make informed decisions about nutrition.

Beyond nutrition, education should also focus on overall healthy lifestyles, including physical activity, stress management, sleep quality, and other factors that influence cancer risk.

By overcoming these challenges and implementing effective education and awareness strategies, it is possible to promote healthy dietary choices and contribute to cancer prevention.

Conclusion

In this chapter, we delved into the dynamic field of scientific research in anticancer nutrition. We explored promising areas of research, examined nutrition-related complementary therapies, and addressed the inherent challenges of this approach. Recent scientific advancements and new perspectives in the field of anticancer nutrition pave the way for more effective approaches and better prospects for prevention and combating this formidable disease.

Encouragement

Introduction

As we come to the end of our journey through the world of anticancer nutrition, it's time to take a pause to reflect, refocus, and find the inspiration needed to continue on the path of health and well-being.

In this chapter, we will explore the importance of personal encouragement, ongoing education, and social support in your journey.

The fight against cancer can be a challenging journey, fraught with obstacles and uncertainties. However, it's essential to remember that you are not alone in this battle. Encouragement, both from yourself and those around you, can be a powerful force in overcoming obstacles and persevering.

We will also delve into the importance of ongoing education and examine why it's crucial to stay informed, continually learn, and rely on reliable sources of information to make informed decisions about your health.

Next, we will look at social and community support. The strength of community and interpersonal relationships can play a vital role in your healing journey. We will explore how to create and nurture a strong support network to accompany you on your journey.

Personal Motivation

Autonomy in health matters is of paramount importance in your motivation to embrace anticancer nutrition. Here's why this concept is so essential for your journey towards better health:

- Personal Responsibility: When you take responsibility for your own health, you become the main actor in your dietary choices and lifestyle. This assumption of responsibility strengthens your commitment to adopting healthier habits because you realize that the results largely depend on you.

- Informed Decision-Making: Autonomy gives you the ability to make informed decisions about nutrition. You can base your choices on reliable information and solid scientific evidence, allowing you to select the foods and strategies that best suit your needs and health goals.

- Personal Satisfaction: When you see the positive benefits of your efforts in anticancer nutrition, it reinforces your self-confidence and personal satisfaction. You are able to measure the progress you have made, which can motivate you to maintain these habits over the long term.

- Independence: Health autonomy empowers you to significantly influence your own health through your dietary choices and lifestyle. This feeling can be a powerful source of motivation.

- Resilience: Autonomous individuals are better prepared to face the challenges and obstacles that may arise when adopting anticancer nutrition. You develop resilience that helps you overcome difficulties and persevere in your efforts for better health.

By embracing your health autonomy, you strengthen your ability to make informed decisions, take responsibility for your well-being, and persevere in your quest for a healthier life. You are at the heart of your own journey towards effective anticancer nutrition.

Continued Education

The Importance of Education

Continued education plays a crucial role in your journey towards effective anticancer nutrition. Here's why it is so important:

- Updating Knowledge: The fields of nutrition and cancer research are constantly evolving. Through continued education, you stay informed about the latest scientific discoveries and the most recent nutritional recommendations.

- Adaptation to Individual Needs: Each of us is unique, with specific nutritional needs. Continued education allows you to adapt your diet based on your age, gender, health status, and other personal factors that are unique to you.

- Addressing Challenges: Daily life can present various challenges that influence your dietary choices, such as busy schedules, budget constraints, or particular food preferences. Continued education helps you find solutions to overcome these obstacles and maintain a healthy diet.

- Prevention of Recurrence: If you have survived cancer, continued education is crucial to prevent disease recurrence. It allows you to maintain a healthy lifestyle and reduce risk factors, thereby contributing to your long-term well-being.

- Motivation and Commitment: Continuous learning can strengthen your motivation by reminding you of the deep reasons why you chose to adopt anticancer nutrition. It can also sustain your long-term commitment by providing you with the knowledge needed to make informed decisions.

By continuing your education in anticancer nutrition, you empower yourself to make informed dietary decisions, adapt your diet to your personal needs, and maintain your commitment to a healthier life. You are at the heart of your own continuous learning, and this can have a significant positive impact on your health.

Reliable Sources of Information

Seeking reliable sources of information on anticancer nutrition is crucial to making informed decisions and avoiding misinformation. Here are some practical tips to help you find trustworthy sources:

- Health Institutions: Websites of national or international health organizations, such as the World Health Organization (WHO) or the Centers for Disease Control and Prevention (CDC), are reliable sources for nutritional recommendations.

- Cancer-Fighting Associations: Organizations like the American Cancer Society or the Canadian Cancer Society provide quality information on nutrition and its link to cancer.

- Scientific Research: Scientific journals, research articles, and academic publications are excellent sources of evidence-based information. They allow you to access the results of serious research.

- Health Professionals: Nutritionists, dietitians, and oncologists are experts in the field of anticancer nutrition. They can provide personalized advice and specific recommendations based on your situation.

- Books and Educational Resources: Books written by nutrition and oncology experts, as well as online courses and other educational resources, can be an excellent source for deepening your knowledge.

- Critical Thinking: It's crucial to exercise discernment when evaluating sources of information. Check if they are based on solid scientific evidence and be wary of sensational or unsubstantiated information.

Setting Realistic Goals

Establishing Personal Goals

Establishing personal goals in anticancer nutrition is a crucial step to succeed in your dietary plan. Here's how you can get started:

- Self-assessment: Begin by reflecting on your current nutrition and health situation. Take the time to analyze your current eating habits, considering your age, gender, and health status.

- Identifying priorities: Identify areas where you would like to make improvements. Perhaps you want to reduce the consumption of certain foods, increase the intake of essential nutrients, or manage your body weight more effectively.

- Specific goals: Define specific and measurable objectives. Instead of saying "I want to eat healthier," opt for concrete goals like "I will consume at least five servings of fruits and vegetables per day."

- Realism: Ensure that your goals are realistic and compatible with your lifestyle, personal constraints, and dietary preferences. Achievable goals are much more motivating.

- Deadlines: Set reasonable deadlines to achieve your goals. For example, decide to reduce your added sugar intake by half over the next three months.

- Tracking and adjustment: Implement a tracking system to assess your progress. This can involve keeping a food journal or using nutrition tracking apps. Be ready to adjust your goals based on your results to keep moving forward.

- These actions will allow you to engage proactively in your journey towards effective anticancer nutrition.

- Importance of Realism

- It is essential to set realistic goals for your journey towards effective anticancer nutrition. Here's why it's crucial:

- Maintaining motivation: Setting achievable goals fosters motivation. Small successive victories encourage further perseverance, as they build self-confidence.

- Avoiding frustration: Overly ambitious goals can quickly lead to frustration and discouragement if not achieved. It's better to aim for attainable milestones to maintain a positive attitude.

- Preventing burnout: Unrealistic goals can lead to mental and physical burnout, which can have a negative impact on your mental and emotional well-being. It's essential to maintain a healthy balance.

- Sustainability: Sustainable nutritional changes are typically those that gradually integrate into daily life. Realistic goals are more likely to become long-term habits.

By encouraging you to set realistic personal goals, we help you adopt a pragmatic approach to anticancer nutrition, thereby increasing your chances of long-term success.

Importance of Realism

It is essential to set realistic goals for your journey toward effective anticancer nutrition. Here's why it's crucial:

- Maintaining motivation: Setting achievable go fosters motivation. Small successive victor encourage further perseverance, as they build self-confidence.

- Avoiding frustration: Overly ambitious goals can quickly lead to frustration and discouragement if not achieved. It's better to aim for attainable milestones to maintain a positive attitude.

- Preventing burnout: Unrealistic goals can lead to mental and physical burnout, which can have a negative impact on your mental and emotional well-being. It's essential to maintain a healthy balance.

- Sustainability: Sustainable nutritional changes are typically those that gradually integrate into daily life. Realistic goals are more likely to become long-term habits.

y encouraging you to set realistic personal goals, we help you opt a pragmatic approach to anticancer nutrition, thereby reasing your chances of long-term success.

ial and Community Support

wer of Social Support

upport is crucial in your journey towards anticancer

imotional support: When undertaking significant nanges in your diet, it's normal to encounter allenges and moments of doubt. The support of your nily, friends, and loved ones can play a crucial role in viding emotional support. They will be there to encourage you, motivate you, and boost your confidence throughout this journey.

- Practical support: Social support can manifest in very practical ways. This can include sharing meal preparation, grocery shopping together, or collectively committing to adopting healthier eating habits at home. This collaboration can ease the transition towards anticancer nutrition.

- Shared responsibility: If several family members or friends are also embarking on anticancer nutrition, it can create a sense of shared responsibility. You will support each other, face challenges together, and celebrate successes collectively.

- Stress reduction: Social support is an excellent way to reduce stress associated with dietary changes. By sharing your experiences and listening to others', you can alleviate concerns and worries. The feeling of not being alone in this endeavor can greatly ease your mind.

By integrating social support into your journey, you enhance your chances of success and create an environment conducive to your success in adopting anticancer nutrition. Remember, you are not alone in this adventure, and the support of your loved ones can make all the difference.

Online Communities

Using modern technology can be an effective way to find social and community support, including:

- Online forums: The internet is full of forums and communities dedicated to anticancer nutrition. It's a place where you can share your experiences, ask questions, and get valuable advice. Joining one of these forums can connect you with like-minded individuals.

- Social media: Social media offers many opportunities to join groups or pages focused on anticancer nutrition. By staying active on these platforms, you stay connected with others who share your interests and goals.

- Mobile applications: You can find mobile applications specially designed to help you track your anticancer diet and connect with others with similar goals. These apps make it easy to track your progress and share your successes.

- Webinars and online videos: Online resources are not limited to forums. You can also find webinars and videos presented by experts in anticancer nutrition. This gives you the opportunity to gain additional insights and hear advice from professionals.

By seeking out and joining online communities, you expand your support network and benefit from the experience and knowledge of others who have committed to anticancer nutrition. This reinforces your commitment and increases your chances of success.

Commitment to a Healthy Life

Adopting anticancer nutrition is not a one-time effort but rather a commitment to your long-term well-being. By choosing to prioritize nutritious foods, maintain a balanced lifestyle, and stay active in your approach, you are investing in your future health. This commitment can help you prevent cancer recurrences and maintain an optimal quality of life.

It's important to keep in mind that every small step you take towards anticancer nutrition matters. Sustainable dietary and lifestyle habits are built gradually, and every positive choice you make contributes to strengthening your overall health.

Personal responsibility is the cornerstone of your success in implementing anticancer nutrition. You have the power to make informed decisions regarding your diet and lifestyle. By actively taking charge of your health, you become the guardian of your own well-being.

It's essential to remember that each person is unique, with individual needs and challenges. By taking responsibility for your health, you can tailor your approach to meet your own needs and goals. This means being mindful of what you eat, how you feel, and how your lifestyle affects your health.

Your commitment to a healthy life and your personal responsibility are the foundations upon which you can build better health and prevent cancer recurrence. By embracing these principles, you take control of your destiny and invest in a healthier, happier future. You have the power to make positive choices for your well-being, and this can make a significant difference in your life.

Conclusion

In this chapter, we delved into the personal and emotional dimension of the fight against cancer. We highlighted the crucial importance of your mindset, determination, and the invaluable support of those around you in your ability to face this complex disease.

Understanding the emotional impact of cancer is essential because it can influence your attitude towards treatment, your level of resilience, and even your physiological response to the disease. Your positive mindset can act as a driving force, enabling you to persevere through the challenges of treatment and maintain an optimal quality of life.

Furthermore, the support of your family, friends, and even specialized support groups can play an invaluable role in your journey against cancer. They can offer a shoulder to lean on, attentive ears to listen to you, and a network of solidarity to help you through tough times.

By addressing this personal and emotional dimension of the fight against cancer, you empower yourself to develop exceptional resilience and approach the disease with determination. This is an essential element for a comprehensive approach to your well-being during this complex period of your life.

Action Plan

Introduction

As our journey through anticancer nutrition comes to an end, it's time to take action and implement all the knowledge and advice you have gained so far.

In this chapter, we will develop a concrete action plan to help you make the necessary changes in your diet, lifestyle, and journey towards optimal health.

Theory and knowledge are essential, but they only truly become valuable when put into practice. Creating an action plan will allow you to transform your intentions into concrete actions, bringing you closer to your health and wellness goals.

Therefore, we will begin by assessing your current diet. You will learn how to analyze your current eating habits and identify areas that need improvement. This essential step will help you understand where you are and where you want to go.

Next, we will explore how to set personalized and realistic goals. We will discuss the importance of setting specific, measurable, achievable, relevant, and time-bound goals to maximize your success.

We will also address time management strategies to integrate dietary and lifestyle changes into your busy daily life. Time is often a precious resource, and we will help you find practical ways to implement your action plan without unnecessary stress.

Finally, we will discuss the importance of continuous monitoring and adjustments. Your action plan is not set in stone, and it may require adjustments along the way. We will provide you with the necessary tools to assess your progress and make the necessary changes to achieve your goals.

This chapter will be your practical guide to implementing everything you have learned during your journey through anticancer nutrition. It will help you transform your knowledge into tangible actions for better health and active cancer prevention.

Evaluation of Your Diet

Self-Assessment

Self-assessment of your diet is the essential starting point for any nutritional modification journey. This step allows you to become aware of what you eat on a daily basis and to determine where opportunities for improvement lie. Here's how to proceed:

- Start by keeping a food journal. Note everything you eat and drink for a few days, detailing portions and times.

- Evaluate the variety of your meals. Are you consuming a wide range of foods, including fruits, vegetables, lean proteins, and whole grains?

- Identify foods rich in essential nutrients and those that are high in empty calories (low in nutrients). This will help you see where adjustments could be made for a more balanced diet.

- Consider your food preferences and personal constraints. This includes your schedule, allergies, cultural preferences, and dietary restrictions.

Dietary Habits

Once you have completed the self-assessment of your diet, it's time to analyze your dietary habits. This step helps you understand your eating behaviors and recognize the strengths and weaknesses of your current diet.

- Identify times when you tend to eat. Is it in response to emotions, such as stress or boredom, or is it related to physical hunger?

- Examine the situations that lead you to make specific food choices. For example, do you often snack while watching television or when you're at work?

- Reflect on your relationship with food. Are you mindful of what you eat, or do you tend to eat automatically?

- Identify foods or food groups that you may be particularly drawn to or those that you often avoid.

Food Journal

Here is an example of a food journal that you can use for the self-assessment of your diet. You can customize it according to your specific needs and the duration you wish to cover, whether it's a few days, a week, or more.

Name: [Your Name]

Start Date: [Start Date of Self-Assessment]

End Date: [End Date of Self-Assessment]

Day 1: [Date]

- Breakfast:
    - [Time]: [Foods consumed]
    - [Time]: [Foods consumed]
- Morning Snack:
    - [Time]: [Foods consumed]
- Lunch:
    - [Time]: [Foods consumed]
    - [Time]: [Foods consumed]
- Afternoon Snack:
    - [Time]: [Foods consumed]
- Dinner:
    - [[Time]: [Foods consumed]
    - [Time]: [Foods consumed]
- Evening Snack:
    - [Time]: [Foods consumed]
- Beverages:
    - [Time]: [Beverages consumed, including water]

Day 2: [Date]

- Breakfast:
    - [Time]: [Foods consumed]
    - [Time]: [Foods consumed]
- Morning Snack:
    - [Time]: [Foods consumed]
- Lunch:
    - [Time]: [Foods consumed]
    - [Time]: [Foods consumed]
- Afternoon Snack:
    - [Time]: [Foods consumed]
- Dinner:
    - [[Time]: [Foods consumed]
    - [Time]: [Foods consumed]
- Evening Snack:
    - [Time]: [Foods consumed]
- Beverages:
    - [Time]: [Beverages consumed, including water]

Feel free to add as many days as you'd like to get a comprehensive picture of your diet. Be sure to include all foods and beverages consumed, along with quantities and times of consumption. This will help you identify dietary trends and determine where adjustments can be made for a more balanced diet.

Setting Personalized Goals

Establishing Goals

When it comes to setting personalized nutritional goals, it's essential to consider your specific needs and individual preferences. Here are some steps to help you define goals tailored to your situation:

- Identification of priorities: Identify areas where you would like to make improvements. Perhaps you want to reduce your intake of added sugar, increase your fiber intake, or incorporate more vegetables into your meals.

- Specific goals: Once you have identified your priorities, set specific and measurable nutritional goals. Avoid vague goals like "eating healthier" and instead opt for goals such as "eating at least five servings of fruits and vegetables per day" or "reducing my soda consumption to one glass per week."

- Adaptation to your lifestyle: Ensure that your goals are adapted to your lifestyle. They should be realistic and achievable, taking into account your schedule, personal constraints, and dietary preferences. Overly ambitious goals can be discouraging.

- Deadlines: Set reasonable deadlines to achieve your goals. For example, you could give yourself three months to reduce your added sugar consumption by half.

Planning Achievable Steps

Once you have defined your nutritional goals, planning achievable steps is essential for successfully achieving them. Here's how to proceed:

- Break down your goals into steps: Take each goal and break it down into smaller, achievable steps. For example, if your goal is to eat more vegetables, one step could be to include a serving of vegetables with every meal.

- Establish an action plan: For each step, develop a specific action plan. Determine how you will incorporate this step into your daily life, what resources you will need, and how you will track your progress.

By following these steps, you will be able to set personalized nutritional goals and plan achievable steps to reach them. This will help you adopt a healthier diet progressively and sustainably.

Time Management Strategies

Meal Planning

Meal planning is an essential strategy for saving time in the kitchen and maintaining an anticancer diet. Here's why it's important and some tips to help you put it into practice:

Importance of Meal Planning

- Time-saving: Meal planning allows you to save time by avoiding the need to decide what to eat every day and by shopping more efficiently.

- Portion control: By planning your meals in advance, you have more control over the portions you consume, which can be important for maintaining a healthy body weight.

- Balanced food choices: You can ensure that your meals are nutritionally balanced by including a variety of nutrient-rich foods.

- Waste reduction: Meal planning helps reduce food waste by efficiently using the ingredients you have on hand.

Tips for Meal Planning

- Establish a weekly menu: Take the time to plan your meals for the upcoming week. Choose healthy and balanced recipes, taking into account your dietary preferences.

- Make a shopping list: Once you have established your menu, make a shopping list based on the ingredients you will need. This will save you unnecessary trips to the supermarket.

- Prepare batch meals: Take advantage of your free time to prepare large quantities of meals that you can reheat when you're pressed for time. This can include soups, stews, salads, or dishes with whole grains.

- Use simple recipes: Opt for simple and quick-to-prepare recipes during the week. There are many healthy recipes that require only a few ingredients and minimal preparation time.

- Invest in airtight containers: Having airtight containers of various sizes allows you to conveniently store leftovers and take them with you for lunch.

- Experiment with takeout meals: If you know you'll be on the go, explore healthy takeout meal options, such as prepared salads, quinoa bowls, or vegetable wraps.

Tips for Quick and Healthy Meals

Even with a busy schedule, it is possible to prepare quick and healthy meals. Here are some tips to help you maintain an anticancer diet even when you're pressed for time:

- Plan simple meals: Opt for simple and quick-to-prepare meals, such as composed salads, bowls of grilled vegetables, or sandwiches filled with fresh vegetables.

- Use pre-prepared ingredients: Save time by using pre-prepared ingredients, such as pre-cut vegetables, canned legumes, or precooked chicken.

- Prepare smoothies: Smoothies can be prepared in minutes and are a healthy option for breakfast or a quick snack. Use green vegetables, fruits, proteins, and seeds for a balanced meal.

- Cook in bulk: When you have free time, prepare extra portions of your favorite dishes and freeze them. This way, you'll always have healthy meals on hand.

- Keep healthy snacks on hand: Have healthy snacks readily available, such as nuts, seeds, fresh fruits, or cut vegetables, to avoid giving in to less healthy temptations.

- Use a pressure cooker: Electric pressure cookers are ideal for quickly preparing meals. They allow you to cook food faster while preserving their flavor and nutrients.

By following these time management strategies, you can maintain an anticancer diet even in a busy schedule. Meal planning and quick, healthy meals will allow you to take care of your health without compromising your lifestyle.

Monitoring and Adjustments

Regularly monitoring your anticancer meal plan and adjusting your goals accordingly is essential for long-term success. Here's why it's so important for you:

- Continuous evolution: Your body changes over time, whether due to age, physical activity, or other factors. Your nutritional needs may also evolve. Therefore, it's crucial to stay attentive to these changes to ensure that your diet remains suitable.

- Self-observation: Continue to observe yourself carefully. Pay particular attention to your energy levels, mood, and any signs of changes in your health. If you notice variations, it may indicate that it's time to make adjustments to your plan.

- Professional consultation: Remember to regularly consult with a healthcare professional or nutritionist. They can help you evaluate your health, adjust your plan based on your goals and current health status, and provide personalized advice.

- Setting new goals: When you achieve your initial goals, set yourself new challenges. Perhaps you want to increase your consumption of beneficial foods or maintain a healthy body weight. Having new goals motivates you to continue progressing.

- Adaptation to circumstances: Life can be unpredictable. Periods of stress, frequent travel, or special occasions can influence your food choices. Learn to adjust your plan based on these circumstances while keeping your long-term goals in mind.

By following these steps and adapting your plan over time, you increase your chances of maintaining an effective anticancer diet and preserving your health in the long term.

Conclusion

In this chapter, we have developed a roadmap for an effective and achievable anticancer diet. We have examined how to evaluate your current diet, set personalized goals, manage your time effectively, track your progress, and implement the nutritional strategies you have acquired throughout this book. You now have the tools necessary to create an action plan specific to your needs, integrating healthy food choices and anticancer lifestyle habits into your daily life.

Commitment to an anticancer nutrition goes beyond knowledge but translates into consistent and sustainable actions. Your action plan is the catalyst for your transformation towards a healthier and more resilient life, resistant to cancer.

Quick Start Guide

Introduction

To help you get started quickly and take immediate steps for your health, we have developed this quick start guide. This guide is designed to streamline your journey towards an anticancer diet and lifestyle. It condenses essential information, provides practical tips, and offers resources to help you make informed decisions from day one.

In this chapter, we will begin by introducing you to the foods you should favor and those you should avoid. You will receive clear guidelines on dietary choices that can support your health and reduce cancer risks. We will also provide practical advice on integrating these dietary changes into your daily life. Change can sometimes be daunting, but we are here to guide you step by step. Next, you will discover a specific dietary guide for different types of cancer. Each cancer may have unique nutritional requirements, and we will help you tailor your diet to meet your specific needs. You will also find information on dietary supplements that may be beneficial.

Finally, you will find simple and healthy recipes to inspire you in your anticancer kitchen.

Foods to Favor and Avoid

Here is a summary of the foods to favor and avoid to reduce the risk of cancer. It is important to note that moderation is essential, even for recommended foods. A balanced and varied diet is key to reducing cancer risks. Additionally, these recommendations may vary depending on the type of cancer and individual needs, so it is advisable to consult a healthcare professional or nutritionist for specific advice tailored to your situation.

Foods to Favor	Foods to Avoid
1. Colorful fruits and vegetables	1. Processed meats (sausages, bacon)
2. Broccoli	2. Deli meats (ham, salami)
3. Cauliflower	3. Red meats
4. Spinach	4. Ultra-processed foods (fast food, snacks)
5. Tomatoes	5. Excessive alcohol
6. Fatty fish (salmon, sardines)	6. Sugary drinks (sodas)
7. Tuna	7. Excess salt

Foods to Favor	Foods to Avoid
8. Extra virgin olive oil	8. Fried foods
9. Berries (blueberries, raspberries)	9. Chips
10. Nuts (almonds, cashews)	10. Cakes and industrial pastries
11. Flaxseeds	11. Grilled beef at high temperatures
12. Beans and legumes	12. Foods high in added sugar
13. Whole grains (oats, quinoa)	13. Fatty dairy products
14. Turmeric	14. Refined grains (white bread, pasta)
15. Ginger	15. Butter
16. Green tea	16. Hydrogenated margarine
17. Garlic	17. Palm oil
18. Red bell peppers	18. French fries
19. Carrots	19. Chicken nuggets
20. Pomegranate	20. Snack crackers

Foods to Favor	Foods to Avoid
21. Oranges	21. High-fat ice cream
22. Chia seeds	22. Whipped cream in a can
23. Red grapes	23. High-fat frozen prepared meals
24. Sweet potatoes	24. Candies
25. Avocados	25. Donuts

Practical Tips

Prioritize fresh and unprocessed foods.

Avoid overcooking, as it can degrade nutrients.

Drink an adequate amount of water throughout the day.

Dietary Guidelines by Cancer Type

Each type of cancer may react differently to certain types of foods, nutrients, and lifestyles. Here are some examples of specific suggestions for common types of cancer:

Breast Cancer

- Encourage consumption of cruciferous vegetables like broccoli, cauliflower, and spinach, which contain beneficial compounds for breast health.

- Limit alcohol consumption, as it has been associated with an increased risk of breast cancer.

- Opt for lean protein sources such as chicken and fish rather than processed meats.

Colon Cancer

- Favor a diet rich in fiber from vegetables, fruits, and whole grains to maintain colon health.

- Limit consumption of red meats and processed meats, as they are associated with an increased risk of colon cancer.

- Drink enough water to avoid constipation, a risk factor for colon cancer.

Prostate Cancer

- Consume foods rich in lycopene, such as cooked tomatoes, which may have a protective effect on the prostate.

- Incorporate omega-3 fatty acids from fatty fish like salmon, which may be beneficial for the prostate.

- Limit consumption of high-fat dairy products, as they may be linked to an increased risk of prostate cancer.

Lung Cancer

- Avoid tobacco smoke, which is the leading cause of lung cancer.

- Consume antioxidant-rich foods such as berries and leafy green vegetables to help protect lung cells.

- Avoid fried and high-saturated fat foods, which may increase the risk of lung cancer.

Ovarian Cancer

- Favor a diet rich in cruciferous vegetables, fiber, and vitamin D-rich foods.

- Avoid processed and sugary foods, as they may influence the risk of ovarian cancer.

- Maintain a healthy weight, as obesity can be a risk factor.

These suggestions are general guidelines, and it is essential to consult with a healthcare professional or oncology nutritionist for personalized advice. Each cancer case is unique, and nutritional needs may vary depending on the stage of the disease, ongoing treatment, and other individual factors. Regular medical follow-up is crucial for cancer management and adjusting the diet accordingly.

Dietary Supplements

Some supplements can be beneficial. Here are some commonly recommended dietary supplements as part of anticancer nutrition:

- Vitamin D: It plays a key role in regulating the immune system and may help reduce the risk of certain types of cancer.

- Vitamin C: A potent antioxidant that can help protect cells against oxidative damage.

- Vitamin E: Another antioxidant that can help strengthen the immune system.

- Selenium: A mineral that may have a protective effect against certain types of cancer.

- Zinc: Important for immune system function and overall health.

- Omega-3 fatty acids: They may help reduce inflammation and maintain cardiovascular health.

- Turmeric (curcumin): It has anti-inflammatory and antioxidant properties.

- Quercetin: A flavonoid found in many fruits and vegetables that may have anticancer properties.

- Resveratrol: A compound found in red wine, grapes, and nuts, which may have beneficial health effects.

- Probiotics: They can help maintain the balance of gut flora, which is linked to immune system health.

Before taking dietary supplements, it is essential to consult with a healthcare professional or nutritionist. They can assess your individual needs, advise you on appropriate dosages, and ensure they do not interact with any other medications you may be taking. A balanced diet remains the foundation of anticancer nutrition.

Easy 2 or 3-Ingredient Anticancer Recipes

Here are 20 simple anticancer recipes made with only 2 or 3 ingredients each:

Spinach and Strawberry Salad

- Ingredients: Fresh spinach, strawberries, balsamic vinaigrette.

- Preparation: Mix spinach and strawberries, then drizzle with balsamic vinaigrette.

Grilled Lemon Salmon

- Ingredients: Salmon, lemon, salt.

- Preparation: Season salmon with salt, then grill with fresh lemon juice.

Kale Avocado Salad

- Ingredients: Kale, avocado, lemon juice.
- Preparation: Massage kale with lemon juice and add avocado chunks.

Garlic Sauteed Broccoli

- Ingredients: Broccoli, garlic, olive oil.
- Preparation: Saute broccoli in olive oil with minced garlic.

Banana Spinach Smoothie

- Ingredients: Banana, spinach, water.
- Preparation: Blend banana, spinach, and water for a nutritious smoothie.

Rosemary Roasted Chicken

- Ingredients: Chicken breast, rosemary, salt.
- Preparation: Season chicken with rosemary and salt, then roast.

Basil Tomatoes

- Ingredients: Tomatoes, fresh basil, olive oil.
- Preparation: Slice tomatoes, add fresh basil, and drizzle with olive oil.

Baked Sweet Potatoes

- Ingredients: Sweet potatoes, olive oil, rosemary.
- Preparation: Chop sweet potatoes, drizzle with olive oil, sprinkle with rosemary, then bake.

Cucumber Mint Salad

- Ingredients: Cucumber, fresh mint, apple cider vinegar.
- Preparation: Dice cucumber, add chopped mint, and toss with apple cider vinegar.

Spinach Omelette

- Ingredients: Eggs, spinach, cheese (optional).
- Preparation: Beat eggs, add spinach and cheese (if desired), then cook as an omelette.

Grilled Lemon Dill Salmon

- Ingredients: Salmon, lemon, dill.
- Preparation: Season salmon with fresh lemon juice and dill, then grill.

Lemon Beetroot Salad

- Ingredients: Beetroots, lemon, olive oil.
- Preparation: Grate beetroots, add lemon zest and juice, then drizzle with olive oil.

Honey Roasted Pears

- Ingredients: Pears, honey.
- Preparation: Halve pears, remove seeds, drizzle with honey, then roast in the oven.

Turmeric Chicken Skewers

- Ingredients: Chicken, turmeric, olive oil.
- Preparation: Cut chicken into pieces, sprinkle with turmeric, add olive oil, then skewer and grill.

Garlic Sauteed Mushrooms

- Ingredients: Mushrooms, garlic, olive oil.
- Preparation: Saute mushrooms with minced garlic in olive oil.

Strawberry Spinach Smoothie

- Ingredients: Strawberries, spinach, water.
- Preparation: Blend strawberries and spinach with water for a healthy smoothie.

Cinnamon Roasted Sweet Potatoes

- Ingredients: Sweet potatoes, cinnamon, olive oil.
- Preparation: Chop sweet potatoes, sprinkle with cinnamon, drizzle with olive oil, then roast.

Orange Carrot Salad

- Ingredients: Carrots, orange juice, sesame seeds.

- Preparation: Grate carrots, add fresh orange juice, and sesame seeds for a colorful salad.

Paprika Roasted Chickpeas

- Ingredients: Canned chickpeas, paprika, olive oil.

- Preparation: Season chickpeas with paprika, drizzle with olive oil, then roast in the oven.

Avocado Grapefruit Salad

- Ingredients: Avocado, grapefruit, fresh mint.

- Preparation: Dice avocado and grapefruit, add chopped fresh mint for a refreshing salad.

These simple recipes are rich in beneficial nutrients for health and can contribute to an anticancer diet. Feel free to customize them according to your preferences.

Comforting Recipes During Treatments

Some comforting recipes can be particularly beneficial during cancer treatments due to their soft texture and ease of consumption. Here are 20 comforting recipes to consider:

Chicken Noodle Soup

- Ingredients: Diced cooked chicken, chicken noodle, low-sodium chicken broth, tender vegetables (carrots, celery), salt and pepper.

- Preparation: Cook noodles in broth, add cooked chicken and tender vegetables for a nutritious soup.

Rice Pudding

- Ingredients: Short-grain rice, milk, sugar, vanilla.

- Preparation: Cook rice in milk with sugar and vanilla to create a creamy dessert.

Mashed Potatoes

- Ingredients: Potatoes, milk, butter, salt.

- Preparation: Mash cooked potatoes with milk, butter, and salt for a smooth mash.

Creamy Oatmeal Porridge

- Ingredients: Oats, milk, honey or maple syrup, sliced bananas.

- Preparation: Cook oats in milk, add honey or maple syrup and banana slices for extra sweetness.

Butternut Squash Puree

- Ingredients: Butternut squash, vegetable broth, butter, salt and pepper.

- Preparation: Cook squash in broth, then mash with butter, salt, and pepper for a velvety puree.

Homemade Applesauce

- Ingredients: Apples, cinnamon, sugar (optional).
- Preparation: Cook apples with cinnamon and sugar (if desired) to create a sweet and soft applesauce.

Banana Yogurt Smoothie

- Ingredients: Banana, Greek yogurt, honey.
- Preparation: Blend banana with Greek yogurt and honey for a creamy smoothie.

Chicken Meatballs with Sauce

- Ingredients: Ground chicken meatballs, sweet sauce (such as apricot sauce).
- Preparation: Cook chicken meatballs and drizzle with sauce for a tasty option.

Berry Oatmeal

- Ingredients: Oatmeal, frozen berries, honey.
- Preparation: Add frozen berries to cooked oatmeal and drizzle with honey for added flavor.

Avocado Spread

- Ingredients: Ripe avocado, lemon juice, salt, pepper, toasted bread.

- Preparation: Mash avocado with lemon juice, salt, and pepper, then spread on toasted bread.

Carrot Ginger Mash

- Ingredients: Carrots, grated fresh ginger, vegetable broth, salt, pepper.
- Preparation: Cook carrots in vegetable broth, then blend with grated ginger, salt, and pepper for a flavorful mash.

Broccoli Velouté

- Ingredients: Broccoli, potatoes, vegetable broth, onion, salt, pepper.
- Preparation: Cook broccoli and potatoes in broth with onion, then blend for a soothing velouté.

Mild Chicken Curry

- Ingredients: Chicken pieces, coconut milk, mild curry paste, diced sweet potatoes, chickpeas (optional).
- Preparation: Cook chicken with coconut milk, curry paste, sweet potatoes, and chickpeas for a tasty and nourishing dish.

Creamy Avocado Pasta

- Ingredients: Pasta (of your choice), ripe avocado, lemon, sour cream (or vegan alternative), salt, pepper.

- Preparation: Blend avocado with lemon juice, sour cream (or alternative), and season for a creamy sauce to mix with pasta.

Vegetable Stew

- Ingredients: Assorted vegetables (carrots, zucchini, leeks), lentils, vegetable broth, thyme, salt, pepper.
- Preparation: Cook vegetables and lentils in broth with thyme, salt, and pepper for a nourishing stew.

Antioxidant Green Smoothie

- Ingredients: Spinach, banana, green apple, coconut water.
- Preparation: Blend spinach, banana, green apple, and coconut water for an antioxidant-rich smoothie.

Creamy Scrambled Eggs

- Ingredients: Eggs, milk (or vegan alternative), butter (or vegan alternative), chopped chives, salt, pepper.
- Preparation: Scramble eggs with milk, butter, and chopped chives for creamy eggs.

Cheesy Zucchini Gratin

- Ingredients: Zucchini, grated cheese (of your choice), sour cream (or vegan alternative), salt, pepper, nutmeg.

- Preparation: Slice zucchini, add grated cheese, sour cream, salt, pepper, and nutmeg, then gratinate for a comforting gratin.

Mixed Berry Chia Pudding

- Ingredients: Chia seeds, milk (or vegan alternative), mixed berries, maple syrup or honey.
- Preparation: Mix chia seeds with milk and mixed berries, sweeten with maple syrup or honey, then refrigerate for a healthy pudding.

Banana Nut Bread

- Ingredients: Mashed ripe bananas, flour, eggs (or vegan substitute), chopped nuts, baking soda, cinnamon, honey (optional).
- Preparation: Mix bananas, flour, eggs (or substitute), nuts, baking soda, cinnamon, and honey (if desired), then bake for delicious banana bread.

These recipes are designed to be gentle on the stomach and easy to digest, which can be comforting during cancer treatments. Remember to consult with your healthcare professional or a nutritionist to ensure these recipes are suitable for your personal situation.

Monthly Meal Plan

Here is an example of a monthly meal plan that can help you maintain a light and balanced diet throughout the month. This plan is designed to provide a variety of nutrients and flavors, incorporating foods rich in vitamins, minerals, and antioxidants. Remember to drink enough water throughout the day and to have healthy snacks, such as nuts, fruits, or vegetables, between meals if needed. You can customize these menus according to your dietary preferences and nutritional needs. The goal is to benefit from a wide range of essential nutrients for your health.

Day 1

- Breakfast: Spinach, banana, and avocado smoothie.
- Lunch: Quinoa salad with grilled vegetables and chicken.
- Dinner: Grilled salmon with steamed broccoli.

Day 2

- Breakfast: Greek yogurt with berries and nuts.
- Lunch: Grilled vegetable and hummus sandwich on whole wheat bread.
- Dinner: Sautéed tofu with Asian vegetables.

Day 3

- Breakfast: Whole wheat bread with almond butter and apple slices.
- Lunch: Lentil and vegetable soup.
- Dinner: Roast chicken with asparagus and quinoa.

Day 4

- Breakfast: Mushroom and spinach omelette.
- Lunch: Chickpea salad with fresh vegetables.
- Dinner: Grilled white fish with green beans.

Day 5

- Breakfast: Berry, oatmeal, and almond milk smoothie.
- Lunch: Cucumber and tomato salad with tuna.
- Dinner: Roasted vegetables with quinoa.

Day 6

- Breakfast: Whole wheat bread with cottage cheese and kiwi slices.
- Lunch: Turkey and vegetable wrap in a whole wheat tortilla.
- Dinner: Grilled tuna steak with sautéed spinach.

Day 7

- Breakfast: Oatmeal with nuts and honey.
- Lunch: Chicken Caesar salad.
- Dinner: Grilled tofu with Mediterranean vegetables.

Day 8

- Breakfast: Strawberry, banana, and almond milk smoothie.
- Lunch: Brown rice salad with vegetables and shrimp.
- Dinner: Salmon fillet with asparagus.

Day 9

- Breakfast: Whole wheat bread with peanut butter and mango slices.
- Lunch: Pea and vegetable soup.
- Dinner: Roast chicken with broccoli.

Day 10

- Breakfast: Tomato and bell pepper omelet.
- Lunch: Quinoa salad with grilled vegetables and feta cheese.
- Dinner: Baked tilapia with brown rice.

Day 11

- Breakfast: Muesli with apple pieces and nuts.
- Lunch: Grilled chicken wrap with crunchy vegetables and yogurt.
- Dinner: Vegetable curry with coconut milk and basmati rice.

Day 12

- Breakfast: Green smoothie with spinach, banana, and almond milk.

- Lunch: Quinoa salad with black beans, corn, and cilantro.

- Dinner: Baked white fish in parchment paper with vegetables.

Day 13

- Breakfast: Whole wheat bread with avocado mash and scrambled eggs.

- Lunch: Red lentil and vegetable soup.

- Dinner: Lemon chicken with asparagus and brown rice.

Day 14

- Breakfast: Greek yogurt with berries and almonds.

- Lunch: Kale salad with apples, walnuts, and grilled chicken.

- Dinner: Salmon steak with dill sauce and roasted vegetables.

Day 15

- Breakfast: Berry, oatmeal, and yogurt smoothie.

- Lunch: Turkey wrap with crunchy vegetables and avocado.

- Dinner: Sautéed tofu with Asian vegetables and brown rice.

Day 16

- Breakfast: Oatmeal with almonds and peach slices.
- Lunch: Greek salad with fresh vegetables, feta cheese, and olives.
- Dinner: Trout fillet with quinoa and broccoli.

Day 17

- Breakfast: Whole wheat bread with peanut butter and banana slices.
- Lunch: Chickpea soup with vegetables.
- Dinner: Grilled chicken with Mediterranean vegetables and couscous.

Day 18

- Breakfast: Mushroom and spinach omelet.
- Lunch: Quinoa salad with grilled vegetables and shrimp.
- Dinner: Cod baked with herb crust and asparagus.

Day 19

- Breakfast: Berry, oatmeal, and yogurt smoothie.
- Lunch: Chicken Caesar salad with grilled chicken.

- Dinner: Grilled salmon with asparagus and quinoa.

Day 20

- Breakfast: Whole wheat bread with peanut butter and mango slices.
- Lunch: Tuna and vegetable sandwich on whole wheat bread.
- Dinner: Sautéed tofu with Asian vegetables and brown rice.

Day 21

- Breakfast: Mushroom, spinach, and feta cheese omelet.
- Lunch: Quinoa salad with grilled vegetables and shrimp.
- Dinner: Roast chicken with broccoli and sweet potatoes.

Day 22

- Breakfast: Green smoothie with spinach, banana, and almond milk.
- Lunch: Turkey wrap with crunchy vegetables and avocado.
- Dinner: Cod baked with Mediterranean vegetables and couscous.

Day 23

- Breakfast: Greek yogurt with berries and almonds.
- Lunch: Kale salad with apples, walnuts, and grilled chicken.
- Dinner: Salmon fillet with dill sauce and roasted vegetables.

Day 24

- Breakfast: Oatmeal with nuts and peach slices.
- Lunch: Greek salad with fresh vegetables, feta cheese, and olives.
- Dinner: Grilled chicken with Asian vegetables and brown rice.

Day 25

- Breakfast: Whole wheat bread with peanut butter and banana slices.
- Lunch: Chickpea soup with vegetables.
- Dinner: Grilled salmon with asparagus and quinoa.

Day 26

- Breakfast: Strawberry, banana, and almond milk smoothie.
- Lunch: Quinoa salad with black beans, corn, and cilantro.

- Dinner: Sautéed tofu with Asian vegetables and brown rice.

Day 27

- Breakfast: Berry, oatmeal, and yogurt smoothie.
- Lunch: Grilled chicken Caesar salad.
- Dinner: Sautéed tofu with Asian vegetables and brown rice.

Day 28

- Breakfast: Whole wheat bread with peanut butter and mango slices.
- Lunch: Tuna and vegetable sandwich on whole wheat bread.
- Dinner: Baked cod with Mediterranean vegetables and couscous.

Day 29

- Breakfast: Mushroom, spinach, and feta cheese omelet.
- Lunch: Quinoa salad with grilled vegetables and shrimp.
- Dinner: Roast chicken with broccoli and sweet potatoes.

Day 30

- Breakfast: Spinach, banana, and almond milk smoothie.

- Lunch: Turkey wrap with crunchy vegetables and avocado.

- Dinner: Salmon fillet with dill sauce and roasted vegetables.

Day 31

- Breakfast: Greek yogurt with berries and almonds.

- Lunch: Kale salad with apples, walnuts, and grilled chicken.

- Dinner: Grilled salmon with asparagus and quinoa.

Conclusion

Throughout the pages of this book, you have gained a deep understanding of the complex relationship between diet, lifestyle, and cancer. You have discovered superfoods that can become your allies in this fight, as well as dietary supplements that can support your health. You have explored various anti-cancer diets and learned to choose the one that suits you best. You have uncovered the role of the microbiome, this invisible ally, and how to take care of it. You have delved into the crucial role of nutrition during cancer treatments, as well as the benefits and risks of calorie restriction and fasting. You have learned to build a fortress against recurrence and commit to a healthy life.

However, beyond the knowledge gained, it is essential to understand that cancer prevention and fight are not just words but actions. It is the implementation of what you have learned that will make the difference. Your action plan, developed in light of this knowledge, will become your roadmap to a healthier and more resilient life against cancer.

Also, remember that medical science continues to advance, opening new perspectives for cancer prevention, diagnosis, and treatment. Stay curious, continue to educate yourself, and remain open to new advances that could improve your health journey. Lastly, do not forget the importance of social support in your journey. You are not alone in this fight, and the strength of the community can be a source of inspiration and resilience.

We hope that the knowledge you have gained here will become the foundation of a healthier life and that you will continue to make informed choices for your well-being. Together, we can strengthen our resistance against cancer and work towards a future where this dreaded disease will become less prevalent. Health is a treasure, and every small step towards a healthier life is a step in the right direction. Keep moving forward, educating yourself, and taking care of yourself. Your health and well-being deserve every effort you put into them.

Resources

Here is a list of books, websites, and other resources that can help you deepen your knowledge of anticancer nutrition, cancer prevention and treatment, as well as promoting a healthy lifestyle:

Books

1. **"Anticancer: A New Way of Life" by David Servan-Schreiber** - This book explores the links between lifestyle, nutrition, and cancer prevention. It highlights strategies to strengthen the immune system and reduce cancer risks.

2. **"The China Study: The Most Comprehensive Study of Nutrition Ever Conducted and the Startling Implications for Diet, Weight Loss, and Long-Term Health" by T. Colin Campbell andThomas M. Campbell II** - Based on a major study, this book examines how diet can influence the prevalence of cancer and other chronic diseases, emphasizing the benefits of a plant-based diet.

3. **"The Cancer-Fighting Kitchen: Nourishing, Big-Flavor Recipes for Cancer Treatment and Recovery" byRebecca Katz et Mat Edelson** - This book offers recipes specially designed to support people with cancer, focusing on nutrition and managing treatment side effects.

4. **"Eat to Beat Disease: The New Science of How Your Body Can Heal Itself" by William W. Li** - This book explores how certain foods can strengthen the immune system and contribute to the prevention and treatment of cancer and other diseases.

5. **"The Longevity Diet: Discover the New Science Behind Stem Cell Activation and Regeneration to Slow Aging, Fight Disease, and Optimize Weight" by Valter Longo** - The author examines how a specific diet can promote longevity and help combat cancer and other age-related diseases.

6. **"Radical Remission: Surviving Cancer Against All Odds" by Kelly A. Turner** - This book explores the stories of people who have survived cancer using unconventional approaches, including dietary changes.

7. **"The Wahls Protocol: A Radical New Way to Treat All Chronic Autoimmune Conditions Using Paleo Principles" by Terry Wahls and Eve Adamson** - The authors share their experience in managing serious illnesses, including cancer, using a diet inspired by the paleo diet.

8. **"The Metabolic Approach to Cancer: Integrating Deep Nutrition, the Ketogenic Diet, and Nontoxic Bio-Individualized Therapies" by Nasha Winters and Jess Higgins Kelley** - This book examines how nutrition, including the ketogenic diet, can be used as an integral part of cancer treatment.

9. **"The Ketogenic Kitchen: Low Carb. High Fat. Extraordinary Health" by Domini Kemp andPatricia Daly** - The book offers recipes and information on the ketogenic diet in relation to cancer fighting.

10. **"Super Immunity: The Essential Nutrition Guide for Boosting Your Body's Defenses to Live Longer, Stronger, and Disease Free" by Joel Fuhrman** - The author explores how optimal nutrition can strengthen the immune system and help prevent cancer and other diseases.

11. **"Cancer-Free: Your Guide to Gentle, Non-toxic Healing" by Bill Henderson and Carlos M. Garcia** - The book provides information on alternative and non-toxic approaches to cancer treatment, including dietary changes.

12. **"The Whole-Food Guide for Breast Cancer Survivors: A Nutritional Approach to Preventing Recurrence" by Edward Bauman and Helayne Waldman** - The book focuses on a nutritional approach for breast cancer survivors, aiming to reduce the risk of recurrence.

13. **"The Cancer Survivor's Guide: Foods that Help You Fight Back" by Neal D. Barnard and Jennifer K. Reilly** - This book provides information on foods that can support the fight against cancer and improve the quality of life for survivors.

14. **"The Essential Guide to Nutrient Requirements" by Food and Nutrition Board, Institute of Medicine** - This book provides guidelines on essential nutrient requirements, which is helpful for understanding how adequate nutrition can influence health.

15. **"The Plant Paradox: The Hidden Dangers in "Healthy" Foods That Cause Disease and Weight Gain" par Steven R. Gundry** - This book highlights foods that can have a negative impact on health and how to avoid them to reduce the risk of diseases, including cancer.

Websites and Organizations

1. **American Institute for Cancer Research (AICR)** - https://www.aicr.org/ - AICR provides resources on cancer prevention through diet, nutrition, and lifestyle. The site offers advice, recipes, and information on ongoing research.

2. **World Cancer Research Fund (WCRF)** - https://www.wcrf.org/ - WCRF focuses on research related to diet, nutrition, and cancer. It provides evidence-based recommendations for cancer prevention.

3. **National Cancer Institute (NCI)** - Nutrition in Cancer Care - https://www.cancer.gov/about-cancer/treatment/side-effects/appetite-loss/nutrition-pdq - NCI offers detailed information on nutrition in relation to cancer care, including managing side effects and promoting healthy eating during treatment.

4. **Cancer Nutrition Consortium** - https://www.cancernutrition.org/ - This organization is dedicated to education and research on nutrition in the context of cancer, providing resources for patients and healthcare professionals.

5. **Cancer Council Australia - Nutrition and Cancer** - https://www.cancer.org.au/about-cancer/causes-prevention/nutrition.html - This site provides information on the relationship between nutrition and cancer, as well as practical advice for healthy eating.

6. **American Cancer Society** - Nutrition for People with Cancer - https://www.cancer.org/cancer/cervical-cancer/treating.html - The American Cancer Society

offers resources on nutrition tailored to people with cancer, covering nutritional needs during and after treatment.

7. **Oncology Nutrition Dietetic Practice Group (ON DPG)** - https://www.oncologynutrition.org/ - This organization focuses on oncology nutrition and provides information for dietitians and healthcare professionals.

8. **The Cancer Nutrition Center** - https://www.cancernutrition.com/ - This center offers personalized nutrition advice for cancer patients, focusing on nutrition as part of treatment.

9. **Susan G. Komen - Nutrition and Breast Cancer** - https://www.komen.org/breast-cancer/survivorship/nutrition-and-breast-cancer/ - This site offers specific information on nutrition for breast cancer survivors.

10. **American Society of Clinical Oncology (ASCO) - Nutrition and Physical Activity During and After Cancer Treatment** - https://www.cancer.net/survivorship/healthy-living/nutrition-and-physical-activity - ASCO provides resources on nutrition and physical activity for people with cancer and survivors.

11. **Cancer Research UK - Diet and Cancer** - https://www.cancerresearchuk.org/about-cancer/causes-of-cancer/diet-and-cancer - This site offers information on the relationship between diet and cancer, as well as tips for healthy eating.

12. **Fred Hutchinson Cancer Research Center - Public Health Sciences - Nutrition Research** -

https://www.fredhutch.org/en/labs/phs/projects/nutrition-research.html - This research center is dedicated to nutrition research and its impact on health, including in the context of cancer.

13. **American Society for Nutrition - Cancer and Nutrition Interest Group** - https://nutrition.org/interest-groups/cancer-and-nutrition-interest-group/ - This organization focuses on the relationship between nutrition and cancer, providing resources for researchers and nutrition professionals.

14. **The Prostate Cancer Foundation - Nutrition and Prostate Cancer** - https://www.pcf.org/about-prostate-cancer/prevention/nutrition/ - This site provides specific information on nutrition in relation to prostate cancer

15. **NutritionFacts.org - Cancer** - https://nutritionfacts.org/topics/cancer/ - NutritionFacts.org offers videos and articles based on scientific evidence to inform about nutrition and its link to cancer prevention.